NUTRITION REVOLUTION©™

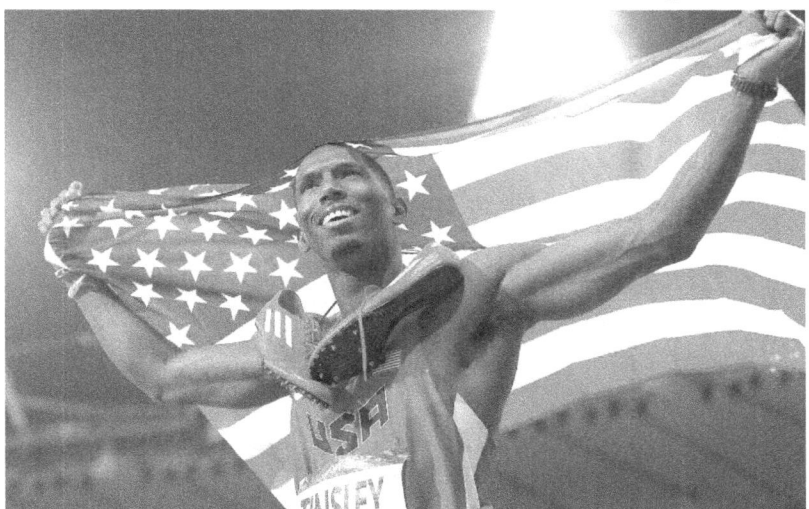

Not a novel. Not fiction.

by
Will David Mitchell
MS, MBA, Nutritionist

Revelation:
The Best Die Young

Doctors

Athletes

Billionaires

Heads of State

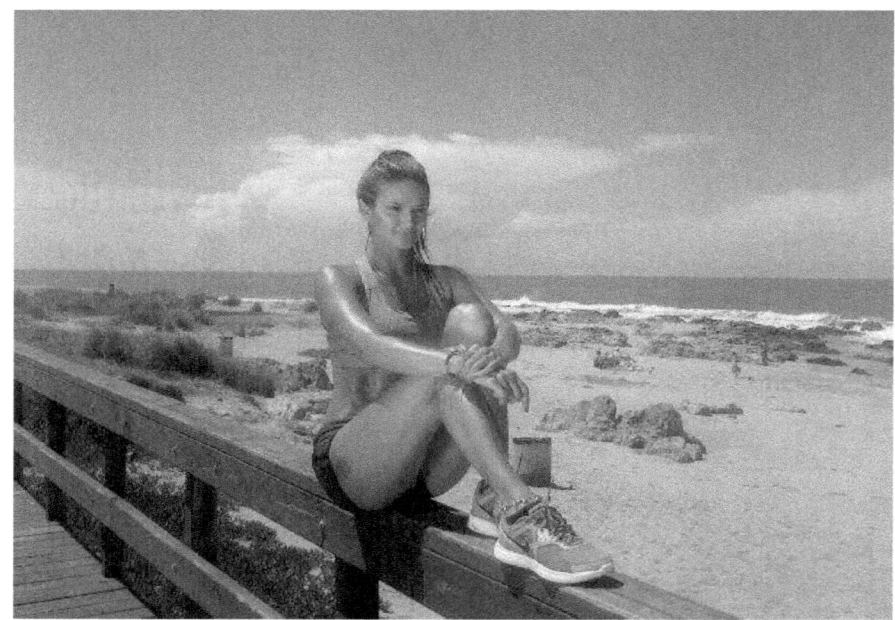

Champion athletes like this track star look and feel exceptionally healthy. Most don't know that exercise without supplementation is dangerous, even suicidal because with every workout, we sweat out the crucial minerals our body needs for long term health.

<u>Do work out</u>. Do keep your body strong but do supplement your diet with the essential minerals. Your body cannot make them and must consume them.

I celebrate our world's athletes. Most books have mandatory blank pages, so I decided to place photos of athletes there instead.

While I do have permission to use the photos of people in this book, I don't have their specific endorsements of its concepts, except for a few like: Theo Ratliff, Drew Pearson, Suzanne Somers, Mike Glen, Gene Nelson, Steve Hess and Marilu Henner.

COPYRIGHT NOTICE

Copyright 2015-2022, Will David Mitchell, All rights reserved.

Only by written permission from the author or publisher, you may review, copy and distribute specified unmodified portions of this work according to the permission given.

This book is in a constant state of revision and updating as new science emerges. The copyright applies to all revisions but not to any original sources that might be owned by others.

All quoted sources are properly attributed in this book.

Published by Intellectual Properties SD, LLC, San Diego.

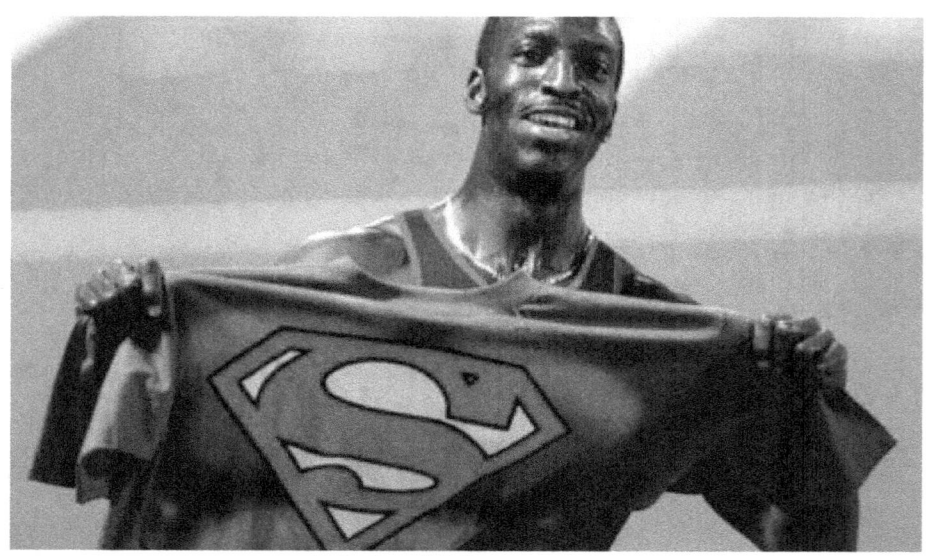

Michael Johnson
Winning the 400-meter race at IAAF Worlds, Greece, 1997.

ABOUT THE AUTHOR

Will David Mitchell is blessed with uncommon energy. At 73 years of age, on a Good Friday, he spent the afternoon running all over a soccer field, showing people how to fly 4-line stunt kites.

After more than three hours, they were winding up their lines, seeking park benches and asking him to go home. He was certain he'd be sore the next day, but wasn't.

The next day, they repeated the playful session. The third day, again, he was not a bit sore and was playing the saxophone as usual in his church's worship band.

He attributes this energy and fitness to the minerals he consumes, quipping that as an USAF pilot three decades ago, he would have been barely moving by Sunday. The minerals weren't available back then.

Then a year later, he repeated exactly the same feat.

David has the gift of writing. In 2011, he decided to write and publish one full-length book a month for a year and did that. All the while, he ran two multi-million dollar corporations and graduated magna cum laude with his second master's degree, this time in business administration. All of that takes unusual energy, especially considering the large amount of time he spends with his family.

Then in October, 2014, he wrote and published two books in ten days, just because someone asked him to teach two courses on those subjects.

He attributes this energy and mentality to the specific, high-quality minerals, vitamins, amino acids and fatty acids he consumes daily. There is only one source for these products: Youngevity.

Generously, he makes Youngevity products available to everyone at Wholesale prices. Retail is more than 42% higher. He pays for your shipping and in most cases your sales tax. He offers a Forever Guarantee on everything he sells. You can find Youngevity products at his official websites, such as:

https://GevityYoung.Com

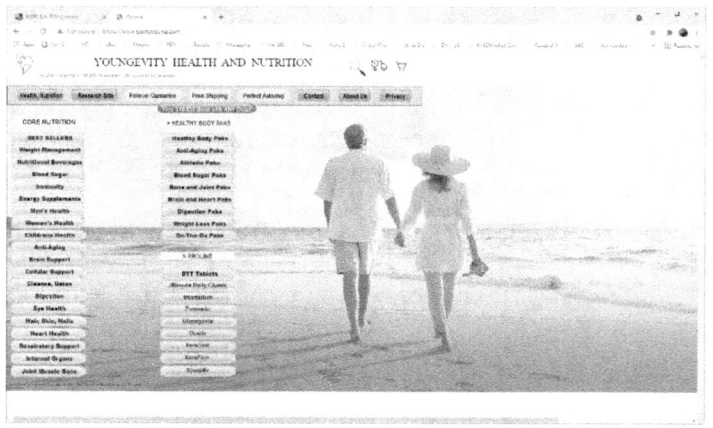

OTHER WORKS BY MITCHELL

The author has written novels, non-fiction and even books that cannot be classified as either!

So, what else is there? He found an affordable way to produce unwritten journals for people. Each one is for one specific person, with their specified title, their name as author and the cover they want. They make excellent, unique $20 gifts, instead of the $6,000 to $12,000 apiece, which they would have cost ten years ago.

Some of David's 150+ websites are:

- https://CleanNovels.Com

- https://MachBooks.Com

- https://WillDavidMitchell.Com

- https://DM1.US Youngevity products

- https://Mktg.Org research on nutrition

Non-Fiction

- The Nutrition Revolution (this book)

- Write Your Own Book (which was written and published in 6 days)

- The New MLM (Business)

- Money Free For The Asking (Negotiation, written and published in 3 days)

- How to (be a) Genius (Solving the impossible)

- Essential Nutrition (With Tank Kobarg)

- Debugging Java (The computer language)

Fiction

Mach Books Series (Spy / Fly Thrillers)

- The Room bOmb

- War, Spying and Flying

- Mach-6

- Kidnapped on the 4th of July

- Maiyan Nation (future space science)

- Maiyan Wars

- Maiyan Lion

- Maiyan Empire

- (three other 'Maiyan' novels plotted)

Dare Series

- Flash Points (The Kobargs are the heroes)

- The Seduction of DoctoRx (Referenced in this book)

- The Wind of God

- Eclipse

- EclipseD

- Total Eclipse

Middle East Series

- How the World Will End (with Cook)

- Sleep Smiling

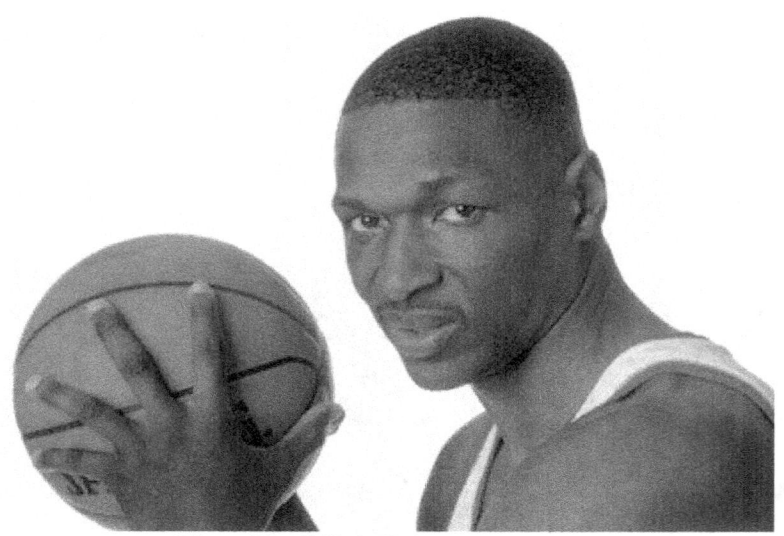

Theo Ratliff, NBA superstar.
Brand ambassador for Youngevity.
Theo credits Youngevity's Rebound™ for restoring his
basketball career after injuries forced him to quit.

DEDICATION

Foremost, I dedicate this work to my personal Savior, Jesus. The first words of the Gospel of John declare that He made us. That includes our DNA, which encodes how our bodies repair themselves on a continuous basis. All we have to do is feed our bodies the raw materials they need.

Second, to my dear wife of 55 years, Carol Mitchell, the finest model for all womanhood to emulate, and also to our children and family.

Also, to our dear friends and fellow laborers in this nutrition crusade, Tank and Patti Kobarg. In 1999, they were nearing an untimely death and we flew to the hospital to pay our last respects to Patti. Tank listened to a tape by our friend Dr. Joel Wallach, called *"Dead Doctors Don't Lie."* Tank arranged an interview with Dr. Wallach and bought the minerals and vitamins that saved both of their lives.

Six weeks later, Carol and I saw them both at a party, many states distant. Convinced, we joined pretty much on the spot.

And to our dear friends, Dr. Joel Wallach and his magnificent wife, Dr. Ma Lan, who founded Youngevity. I can't count the number of lives they have saved; nobody can. Surely the count is deep into the millions.

They are American heroes of the first order.

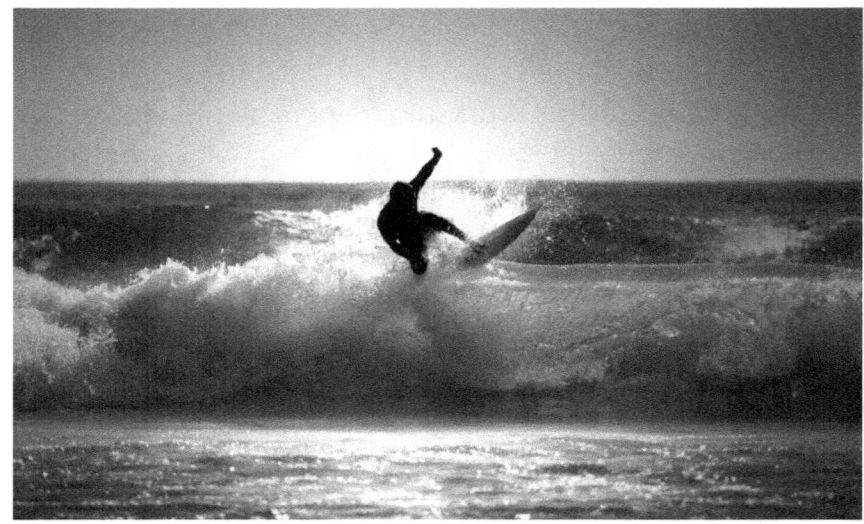

Surfing the molten waters of San Diego in winter

REVISIONS

This is a "Living" book. When you buy a copy, even if you acquire it as a gift, you receive more than that individual copy. You also gain all revisions, for life, free for the asking.

We do need your current email, so we can send new editions to you.

Revisions are important because science is an incremental thing. All science is derivative. It is always in the process of building on itself, in spurts of knowledge. No scientist ever discovers or invents anything without building on the works of others.

For example, a scientist may invent a unique tool that helps other scientists discover something. Even the tool is based on the work of earlier men and women, perhaps metallurgists or machinists, perhaps optical scientists or atomic scientists, perhaps chemists or computer scientists.

Science advances incrementally in the fields of medicine and nutrition also. As new science emerges and as we research new fields, we change this book. Thus we revise it and send you free electronic copies. We want there to be no secrets.

Obviously, we can't revise books that have already been printed but we do offer new editions. Amazon supports our paid Kindle books by sending you free revisions as soon as we release them. They do that automatically. As we revise a Kindle book, Amazon delivers the new one to you in minutes.

Commercially, we sell this book for $34.95 because of the decades of research and experience we've all put into this entire project. It's a huge bargain at that price. It is a master's level course in nutrition, and the full color version is also available. A comparable college textbook costs more than a hundred dollars. This book may well expand to an encyclopedia, in which case the set will cost a bit more.

We won't charge anyone a hundred dollars for one book. You might not buy it and that means you wouldn't reap the benefits of this knowledge. More than anything, we want you to be healthy.

For revisions, write David@Mktg.Org. Leave your name and email address. We'll email you the secret key so you can download the latest version. Legally, we can't send it to you unless you give us permission. Do not worry; we will never share your email address with anyone for any reason.

Check the revision date at the upper left corner of the book cover on the website vs. your book. If we have a newer version available, just download it.

If you don't have a computer, you might go to a library or use a friend's computer and read or download the book. You can print a copy or read it online. That's fine with us. As financing allows, we hope to make audio versions available and will tell you if we succeed.

We'll send you notices of updates and other medical or nutritional news that we uncover. We're bargain hunters and tell you where you can buy nutritional products at the lowest possible prices – usually wholesale – never higher than we pay personally. We ask you to tell us about bargains you find, so we can share the knowledge.

In particular, we pledge to make Youngevity products available at the lowest possible prices (wholesale) and in most cases we can afford to arrange free sales tax out of the 8% rebate Youngevity gives us for spreading the nutritional word. We pay your shipping costs (about 8%) and when possible your sales tax (another 8-11%). We Guarantee Everything Forever.

Just go to **http://DM1.US** to browse or shop at wholesale prices.

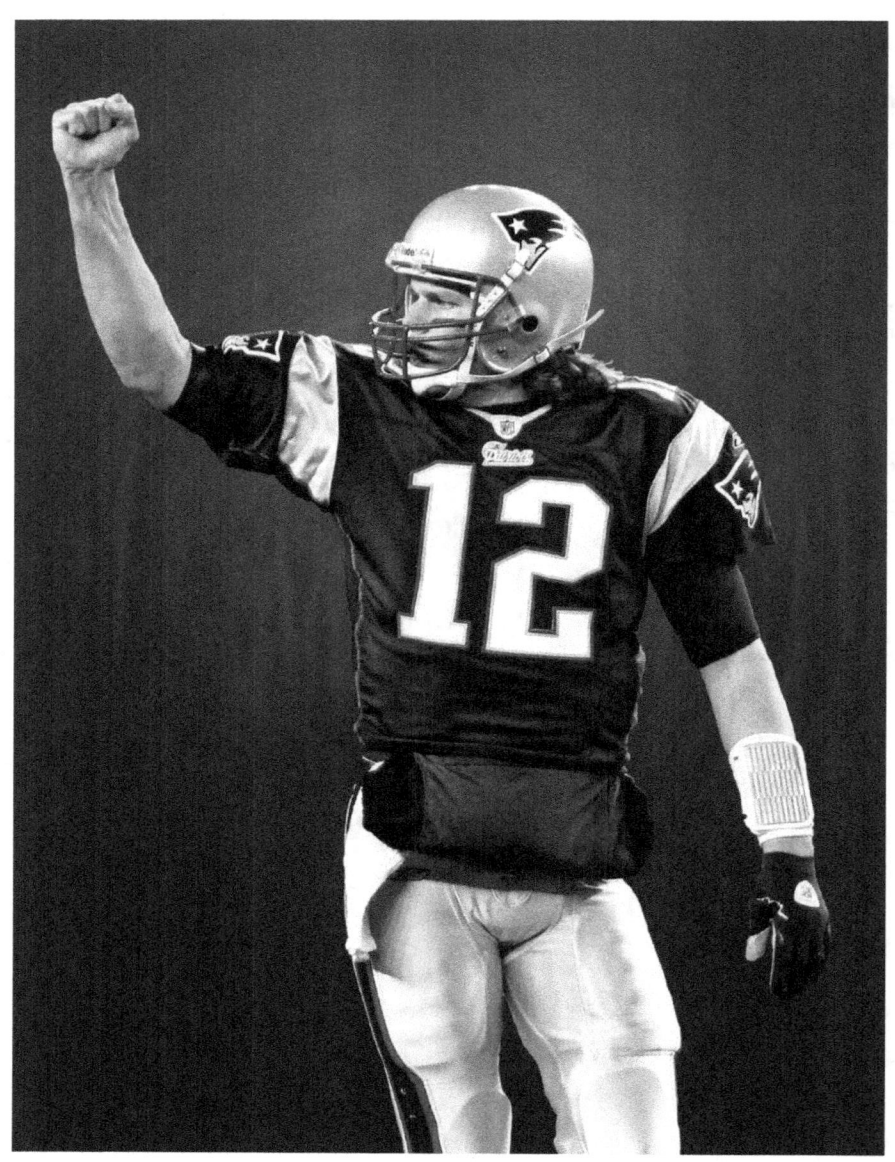

Tom Brady, Seven Time Superbowl Champion
Quarterback, Washington Patriots

TABLE OF CONTENTS

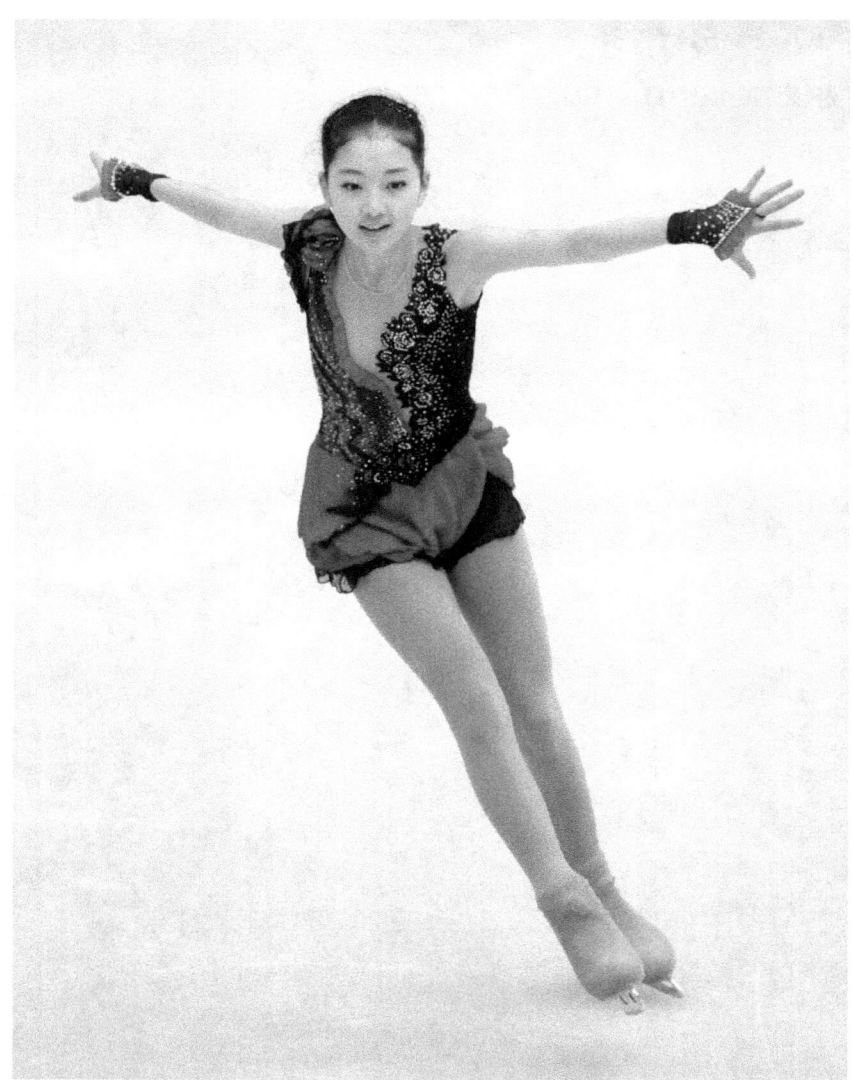

Li Zijun, Ice Dancer

FORWARD

Question: Who's worthy of our dietary trust?

- The government told us to restrict salt because it causes high blood pressure.

  - At last, they admit that's a faulty idea and that **we should salt to taste.** Unfortunately, a huge number of people have developed severe and deadly digestion problems due to insufficient salt to make stomach acid.

  - Two new facts emerged 3/5/15. You can find the whole article later in this book, with references.

    - First, salt is important in fighting infection and inflammation.
    - Second, the overly-low recommended salt intake increases risk of heart attacks by a factor of 2 to 3, especially among people who are already at risk for heart disease.

- The government told us to use antacids to reduce stomach acid.

  - Research has shown that the **problem is too little acidity in the stomach,** allowing bad organisms to flourish and destroy digestive enzymes. They also cause gas and acid reflux. The problem is too little acidity, not too much.

- The government told us to restrict eggs because they cause high cholesterol.

- o Now, they say **eggs are fine** and are a good source of inexpensive protein and it's okay to eat 6-12 a day.

- The government told us to concentrate our diets on grains, using the food pyramid.

  - o Now, they've debunked that idea, inverting the pyramid and saying **meats and beans are far better for us than grains.**

- The government spent untold millions defending the falsehood that selenium is poisonous, and then that selenium is not effective as a food supplement.

  - o A private citizen spent millions of his own money to force the government to admit **Selenium is effective against Prostate, Lung and Breast cancers -- and now, several other cancers.**

- The government said that Omega-3 Fatty Acids are bad for us.

  - o They lost a lawsuit on that issue and have been forced to admit **Omega-3 Fatty Acids promote heart health.**

- The government tried to convince us that GMO foods are safe.

  - o At last, they are begrudgingly admitting that **GMO foods contribute to all manner of diseases**.

- o I read that they are allowing a new GMO Granny Apple to be produced, merely because it resists browning from oxidation! They admit that cooks have added lemon juice to apples for decades, to prevent browning. They don't seem to care that Granny Apples will still oxidize like the rest – but that such spoilage will be hidden from the consumer! Boo, hiss, and rotten apples!

- For 39 years, the government told us to restrict red meat, lobster, shrimp and other foods high in cholesterol.

  - o In 2015, they admitted that **high cholesterol does not cause any form of cardiovascular disease.**

That's not even the half of it. Butter is vindicated over margarine but that story is far from over. Fried foods are still considered okay, despite the carcinogenous nitrites and nitrates forming naturally in the hot oil. Sugar is considered fine for school children despite its effects on teeth and body fat.

If not the federal experts, who should we believe?

Apparently not the government. Their track record isn't good.

In 2015, they admitted that nutrition science 'obviously' needs a lot more research money. In my opinion as a scientist, that clever spin on their failure is hogwash! Nutrition science needs a lot more common sense, not a lot more riches for the researchers. Common sense needs to be more common.

There are a few learned people who have been on the right track all along. They have been preaching:

THE NUTRITION REVOLUTION

1. **Don't restrict salt.** Salt to taste. Your body needs salt and will tell you how much is correct for you because the food will taste right. If your body has too much, salty food will taste bad and you'll avoid it.

2. **Avoid GMO foods.** Nearly all corn is from GMO seed. Ditto for most soybeans and their products.

3. **Eliminate gluten** in the diet, especially from the grains Wheat, Rye, Barley and Oats. Gluten blocks the body's ability to absorb nutrients, all of them, including the vital minerals, vitamins, amino acids and fatty acids you need to thrive.

4. **Eat plenty of eggs and red meat,** so you will have enough cholesterol in your diet to keep your brain and nervous system functioning correctly. Dr. Wallach, Dr. Glidden, I and many others eat 6-10 eggs a day.

5. **Avoid fried food.** It's not so much for the added fat as for the nitrates and nitrites that heat creates in the oil. Frying oil turns rancid almost instantly at high heat and converts into cancer-causing nitrates and nitrites. Some of those chemicals soak into the food. If you're going to fry an egg, at least use butter and low heat. Poaching or boiling is even better.

6. **Cook in butter,** never margarine or other oils. Even olive oil goes rancid in the bottle. It commonly sits for a long time before use and every time you open the bottle, new oxygen enters, making it become rancid.

7. **Consume Omega-3, 6 and 9** essential fatty acids.

8. **Take inexpensive Selenium** to prevent many cancers and other diseases.

9. **Supplement your nutritionally-deficient food** with a total of 90 Essential Minerals, Vitamins, Amino Acids and Fatty Acids.

Such forward-looking people include(d):

- Dr. Joel Wallach
- Dr. Ma Lan
- Dr. Peter Glidden
- Dr. Bernhard Schrauser
- Dr. Richard Renton

I could list 25 others.

These people and other like-minded research scientists, not the Federal Drug Administration (FDA,) nor Big Pharma nor the government, are the kinds of people to follow if you want to "live long and prosper" in great health.

I pause a moment to honor Leonard Nimoy, a fine, prolific and wide-ranging actor and poet. Leonard died quite prematurely yesterday in his Bel Aire home. The whole world has enjoyed his portrayal of Mr. Spock on Star Trek, where he made popular the phrase "live long and prosper".

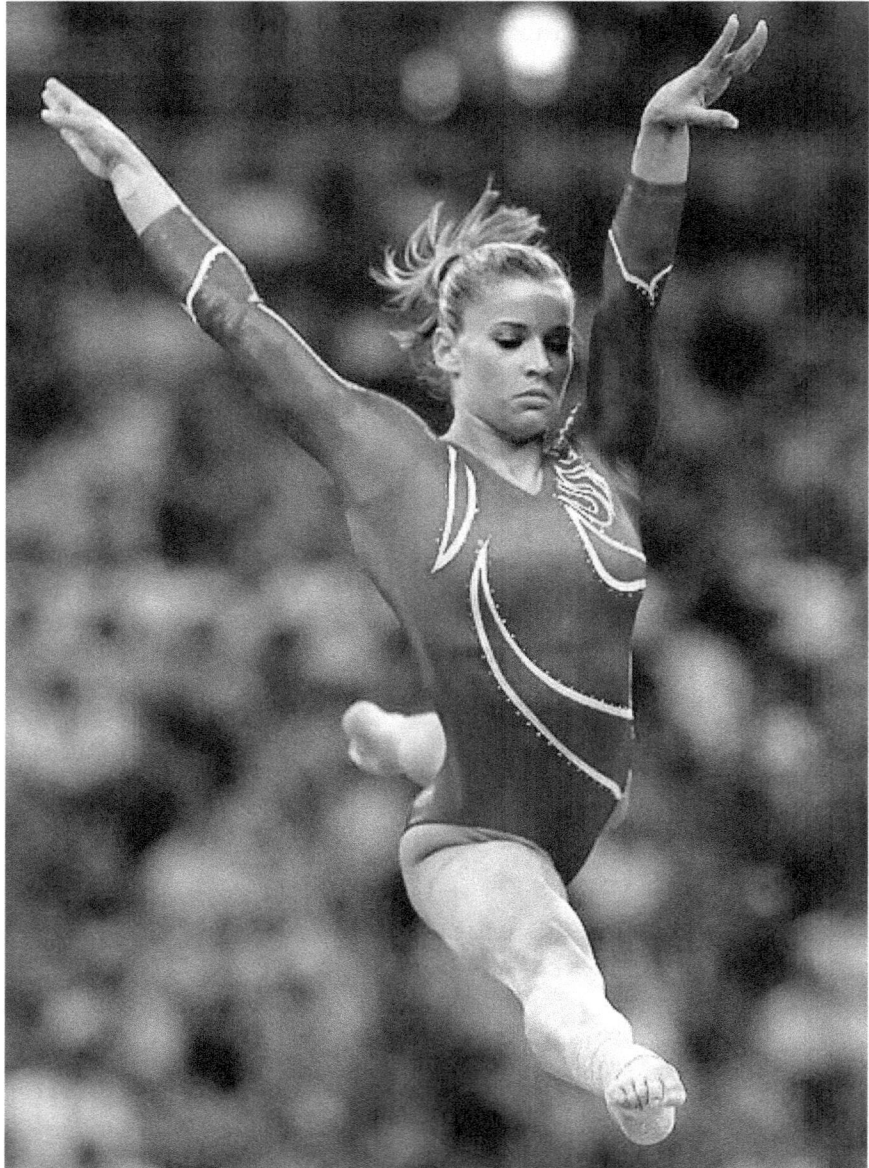

Gymnast above the Balance Beam

MODULE ONE

The Best Die Young

Why do:

- Doctors,
- Professional Athletes,
- Powerful Politicians,
- Billionaires

        die long before their time?

A few gain wisdom and understanding, living long, healthy lives.

> *The Bible says: "If any of you lacks wisdom, you should ask God, who gives generously to all without finding fault, and it will be given to you." James 1:5. New International Version.*

Here are some of those wise, long-lived people:

Art Linkletter, the originator of *"Kids Say The Darndest Things,"* understood wisely. He researched longevity, learned its secrets and made it to age 97.

Bob Hope and George Burns understood it and lived past 100.

Linkletter, Hope and Burns are comedians. The very funny lady Betty White is nearing 100 and working at this writing. Maybe it's related to comedy. Some say laughter is the best medicine.

Most rich, highly trained people don't live long.

No recent, professional athletes have lived to 100. (Ed. One finally did recently. Just one.) Sadly, they die at an average age of around 60. They train and exercise in their youths and throughout their careers. They do punish their bodies but they do it to be strong and remain healthy for longer lives. Instead, they are **more** prone to injury than the rest of us and they die 16-years too early. Their diligence fails to lengthen their lives.

You should exercise but you must supplement your diet with the minerals your body sweats out during workouts. Then, you'll be healthy and long-lived. However, the average couch potato lives longer than the average athlete who doesn't supplement his or her diet correctly.

Athletes who do supplement their diets, live long lives.

Those who don't, just don't.

THE NUTRITION REVOLUTION

Billionaires are remarkably short-lived. They have access to the finest medical treatment. Strangely that doesn't keep them as healthy as the couch potato watching TV and eating junk food. Uncounted wealth couldn't save Steve Jobs recently. The rich die early for the same reason professional athletes do.

Even omitting assassinations from the statistics, **powerful leaders of nations die too young.** We watch young presidents age from TV appearance to TV appearance, almost before our eyes. The reason? It's the same.

So what chance do the rest of us have? Evidently we have a better chance than the rich and famous!

It's an issue that's certainly worth examining. Read on. There's mighty wisdom in the coming pages.

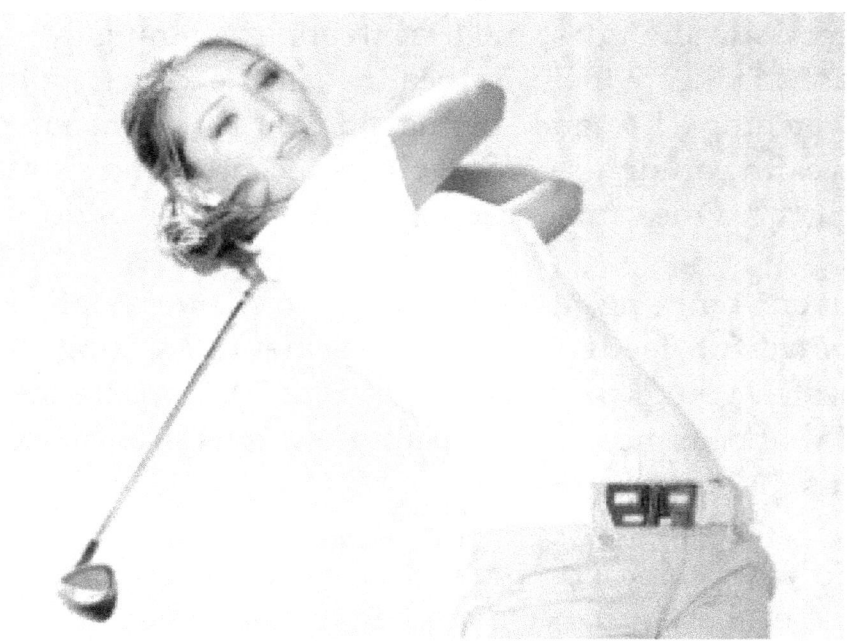

Maiya Tanaka

MODULE 2

The Role of Medicine

Some of the world's best researchers claim that these early deaths have something to do with medicine and I agree.

Here is the counter-intuitive pattern:

Those who can afford the best medicine die young.

Those who can't get it – live longer!

One would think the opposite would be true.

Details

In 2008, the average American lived to an age of 78. As of 2008, the World Health Organization reports that citizens of forty-three countries, whether they were developed nations or not, lived longer than Americans. Look at this list of countries and their average life spans.

Andorra	83.52
Antigua and Barbuda	82.3
Macau	82.27
Japan	82.02
San Marino	81.80
Singapore	81.80
Hong Kong	81.68
Sweden	80.63
Australia	80.62
Switzerland	80.62
France	80.59
Guernsey	80.53
Iceland	80.43
Canada	80.34
Cayman Islands	80.20
Italy	79.94
Gibraltar	79.93
Monaco	79.82
Liechtenstein	79.81
Spain	79.78
Norway	79.67
Israel	79.59
Jersey	79.51
Faroe Islands	79.49
Greece	79.38
Austria	79.21

Virgin Islands	79.20
Malta	79.15
Luxembourg	79.03
Montserrat	79.00
New Zealand	78.96
Germany	78.95
Belgium	78.92
Guam	78.76
Saint Pierre and Miquelon	78.76
European Union	78.70
United Kingdom	78.70
Finland	78.66
Isle of Man	78.64
Jordan	78.55
Puerto Rico	78.54
Bosnia and Herzegovina	78.17
Bermuda	78.13
Saint Helena	78.09
United States	78.00

There we are! That was in 2008 and the USA lagged Andorra, the best nation by 5.5 years.

By 2014, the United States moved up a couple of points to #42. The whole world lived longer too but it was primarily due to better sanitation, not medical advances.

In 2014

People in little Monaco lived to 89.57 years.
People in the USA lived to 79.56 years, worse by more than 10 years!

So in five years, the United States went from

5.5 years behind Andorra, the #1 nation to

10 years behind Monaco, the new #1 nation.

Source: the World Health Organization.

A Principle

Those Who Live Furthest From Good Medicine Live Longest.

Considering smaller cultural groups instead of entire nations, people who live the farthest from 'modern' medicine tend to have the very best longevity on earth.

Often, they are driven to inaccessible areas, such as high in the mountains, by political forces. Such people live far longer than people in the United States do.

Often, their water is polluted by minerals from glacial runoff – called Glacial Milk because it's not clear. Some researchers like Dr. Wallach have found that this kind of mineral pollution is exactly what the rest of us need.

Yeah!

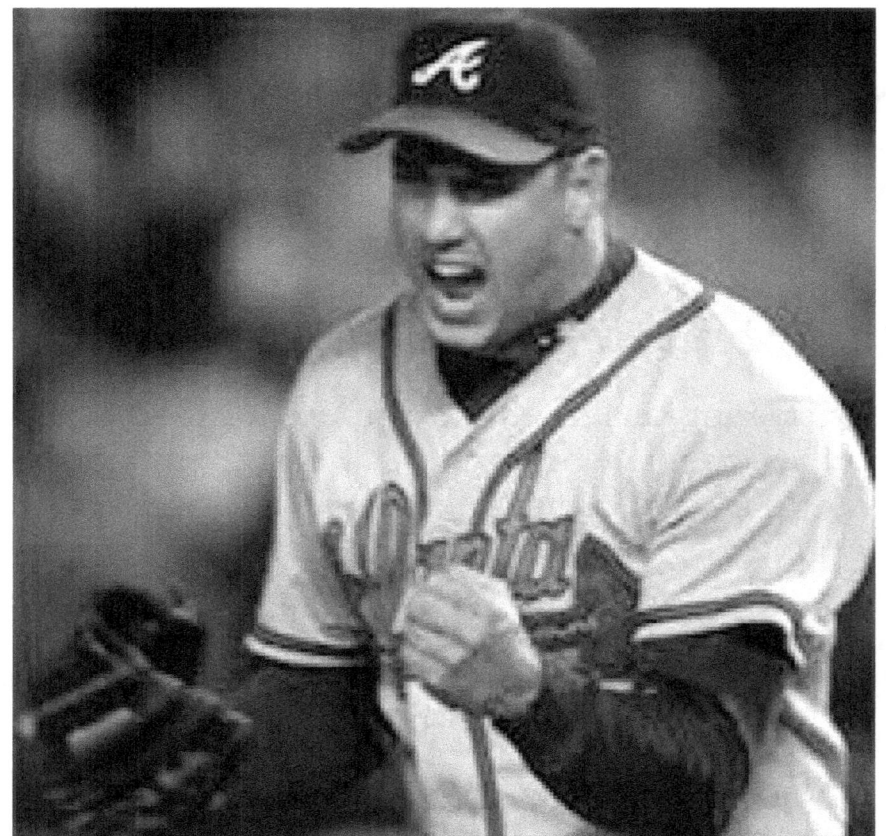

Yeah!

Why Do MDs Die Early?

I have a see-through sign on the rear window of my car, saying:

**DEAD DOCTORS DON'T LIE
FREE CD 858-538-9455**

I get curious tailgaters.

It's okay. I keep sufficient distance from the car in front and let them read.

Occasionally, someone will call on my cell phone while I'm driving, and inquire about the sign.

When I ask where they are, they will say they're right behind me. In California, it's okay to answer or dial out while driving but one can't hold the phone. So, I go to hands-free mode, ask them to do the same and explain to them,

"The reason Dead Doctors Don't Lie is because they are dead."

After sharing an ironic laugh, I explain what the sign means.

The doctors are dead because they follow their own advice. Their longevity is proof positive of how good or bad their advice is.

They die at an average age of 57. Obviously they take their own advice. That proves they are advising their patients poorly.

Here's something astonishing: **Homicide Detectives are the only professionals who live shorter lives than doctors.**

Their statistics are skewed. They make their living by putting themselves in harm's way, such as by surviving gun battles. Worse, they have a high suicide rate.

Source: Wikipedia.

Since the suicide rate of doctors is not very high, that means doctors are Dead Last in terms of longevity.

Before I explain these grim statistics to my caller, I try to find out why they called me. If it's because they are facing a crisis, particularly a medical crisis, the odds are huge that I can help. A lot.

> o Bone and Joint Pain? They can be pain-free in 10 days and free of arthritic symptoms in 3-5 months.

- o Blood Sugar Problems? It usually takes about 60-120 days to bring blood sugar under control.

- o Cancer? Some types disappear quickly, others more slowly. Better longevity is assured.

- o Muscular Dystrophy? High Cholesterol? Alzheimer's?, Lou Gehrig's?, Multiple Sclerosis?, Dementia? All are related. All can be improved or reversed.

- o Dietary diseases and Celiac can be stopped and gradually reversed.

- o Hereditary Diseases simply aren't hereditary after all. We don't get them from our parents (nor from our kids!) Nutrition prevents and fixes them, although the damage can be long-lasting. Prenatal supplementation is a must.

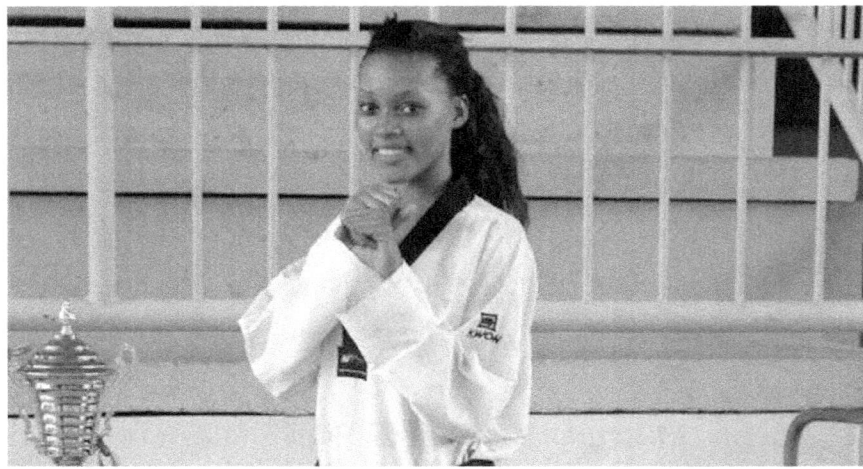

Cynthia Kragve, Taekwondo Champion

If MDs cannot heal us, Who Can?

It's a simple, profound concept. <u>The human body heals itself.</u>

You knew that.

MDs know that.

Everyone knows that.

All you have to do is to help it by providing the essential raw materials. You and your parents have been doing that all of your life. There's almost no medical difference between healing and growing up.

Physicians admit that they can't cure or heal anything. The body heals itself.

1. If they let it.

2. Sometimes they give the healing process a boost by killing off or removing some bad organisms. Excellent.

3. Sometimes they mask symptoms instead of treating the disease. Not so excellent.

4. Sometimes, the symptom-masking drugs they prescribe must be taken for the rest of

one's life. I call that prescribing an addiction.

Two months ago, a physician who's acknowledged locally as the best in his field, admitted it to my wife and me, saying with a smile,

> *"We are addicted to air and water so what's the difference if we become addicted to pain pills?"*

The **massive difference** is that there are no adverse side effects when we breathe air, drink water. He continued with a smile,

> *"Of course, I wouldn't give this to an 18-year old."*

He was only working on her knee.

In other words, he gave us a lot of encouragement, implying that my dear wife isn't going to live much longer anyhow, so what's the difference!

MASSIVE difference.

My dear wife is going to live long and prosper in great health.

The Problem With Prescriptions

Every prescription drug has adverse side effects -- by definition.

That's precisely why it's only administered by prescription. A doctor must monitor the side effects and deleterious problems the drug causes. If there were no side effects, there would be no medical need for it to be prescribed by doctors.

Each time a physician writes a prescription, the patient is trading one set of symptoms for another set of symptoms, called side effects. Hopefully, it's a good trade.

For example, pure water has no side effects. It is not a drug, precisely because it has no side effects. Doctors don't pull out their prescription pads when advising people to drink plenty of water.

Neither do they write prescriptions for air, food or food supplements. It is precisely because these things don't have bad side effects. The effects are all good – when those things are taken within reason. Of course, any good thing is bad when taken to excess.

The body regulates its health in amazing ways we don't appreciate.

- Getting full at a meal is one of them. Our bodies know how much food is right and unless we seduce our palates with sweets and tasty cuisine, our bodies will tell us when to stop eating.

- Using the right amount of salt is another way our bodies are amazing. Our bodies crave salt but not too much. A steak is ruined when the chef puts too much salt on it. That's why we have salt shakers in restaurants. We all need and desire differing amounts of salt. Every farmer and rancher puts out blocks of salt for the cattle to lick. As Dr. Wallach says, nobody tells the cow how many licks to take. The cow knows. So do the deer and other animals that use the salt licks.

  Salt's benefits have been so highly prized by humans in history that it has served as money. The word 'salary' is derived from the Latin word for salt.

Salt does NOT elevate blood pressure. A study saying it did was fatally flawed. That study found a statistically insignificant rise in blood pressure in a small number of individuals Who Already Had Extremely High blood pressure. Even that result was statistically insignificant, meaning the tiny elevation might have been attributed to any number of other factors. For the rest of the population, there was no increase. On the basis of that, the FDA recommended salt restriction!

Source: Dr. J.D. Wallach.

Edible formulations without side effects (such as steak, beans, breakfast, water, salt, silver, minerals, vitamins) are classified as food and are sold without a prescription. Minerals and vitamins are considered food by the law, exactly because they are safe.

In the 1980s and 1990s, pharmaceutical companies tried to get food supplements declared drugs. They wanted to put the food supplement companies out of business and take over. They lost that fight over the side effects issue.

There's a more sinister reason drugs exist. Companies can patent drugs. They can't patent food supplements. They can charge more for patented things.

That's why pharma companies wanted vitamins and minerals to be classified as drugs, so they could patent and restrict them.

This doesn't mean that foods are impotent in the treatment of disease. Silver, listed above, cannot be patented. It <u>has been classified as a food.</u> That means that it doesn't fit under the purview of physicians – despite the fact that it is an effective antibiotic when in colloidal form. Most ionic forms of silver are dangerous and must be consumed with considerable care.

My family uses colloidal silver to knock out respiratory illnesses before they begin. We swallow a spoonful slowly. Most such illnesses begin in the back of the throat and the silver prevents viruses and bacteria alike from reproducing. We use zinc lozenges (not the tiny pills) for the same thing. It works.

Doctors are prescribing silver for viral diseases like Ebola. Although silver is a food, a dozen research teams are reporting good success against Ebola using various ways to deliver silver, such as is used by our acquaintance, Dr. Garcia in Mexico to reverse and eliminate HIV/AIDS in humans. I tested and proved the safety of the electronics used in Dr. Garcia's treatment.

THE NUTRITION REVOLUTION

Dr. Garcia's first human trials were on 500 people. In six weeks 497 had negligible to zero viral count in their bloodstreams. Three died of other causes. His treatment is poised to be released to the world.

Source: Robert Maddux

Since everything that is a drug has side effects, by definition, every drug is dangerous to some significant degree and must be monitored by a physician. If there were no danger, it wouldn't be classified as a drug. That is the law.

Some drugs are far more dangerous than others. At one extreme, heroin and cocaine are famously addictive drugs. They still have a few, very rare medical uses. They dull pain. They dull the mind and prevent it from thinking. They also deteriorate the body. When a patient tries to stop taking them, the withdrawal symptoms ravage the whole body. They are debilitating. They cause such extreme pain that the body may perish, and in any case, the addicts hope they will die.

Other drugs are less 'dangerous' only because they may take a longer time to cause severe or fatal damage. Withdrawal can be equally devastating and deadly. Just watch the TV ads for proof.

- A widely-prescribed class of drugs called statins, for instance, gradually ruins the kidneys. *"Tell your doctor if you have any kidney problems,"* the TV advises on statin commercials.

- Tylenol is the most widely taken and prescribed pain killer. It and its cousins ruin the liver. It may take years but without kidneys, without a liver, the body perishes from very nasty conditions the doctors call diseases.

- TV advertisements are rife with drug ads that list the side effects and then tell you to: *"Ask your doctor if {drug-x} is right for you."*

In other words, try to persuade your doctor to prescribe it, because you know more than your M.D. does about this drug. After all, you saw it advertised on TV, with beautiful people playing badminton or throwing a Frisbee on the beach. Although they're probably actors, they might be taking that drug. The implication is that they are and they have no adverse side effects and that they are cured.

Of course, those side effects won't happen to you – you hope. Reality says they will, universally.

More importantly, you provide income to your doctor. Your MD should honor your request and keep your pay flowing into his or her coffers.

Is that how it should be? Or perhaps should your money pay for the doctor's unbiased opinion?

Yes, that's it. After all, the MD knows that drug exists and has studied its side effects. The drug companies made sure the doctor knows the drug exists.

Perhaps we shouldn't try to bias the doctor. Perhaps Big Pharma shouldn't be allowed to advertise prescription drugs on TV.

I think the word "perhaps" doesn't belong in those last two sentences at all.

- Various other drugs cause diseases of the kidneys, liver, brain, heart, intestines, nervous system – and doctors prescribe those drugs with full knowledge of what they do. Doctors aren't out to kill you. <u>The whole idea is to trade temporary relief for a shortened life.</u>

There is a better way, a safer way, a permanent way. The body heals itself, given even a partial chance.

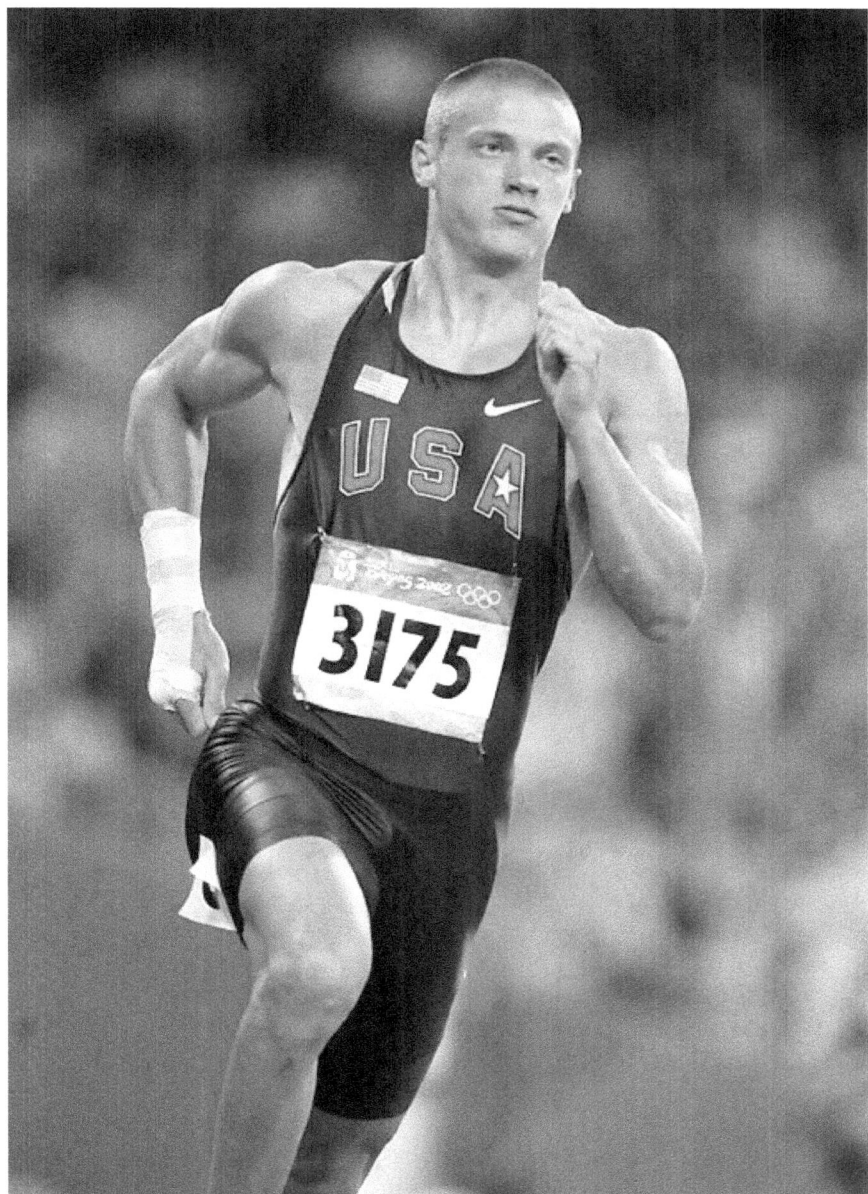

Athletes compete despite injuries.
Earlier, this man broke a bad fall with his right hand and
wrist. Fortunately for him, he was able to make his next run.

MODULE 3

The Nutrition Connection

The body wants to heal itself. The only way to stall this <u>miracle of healing</u> is to starve the body of the 95 nutrients it needs for life. Remove any of those essential nutrients and the body sickens and dies.

Sometimes the sickening process takes minutes, as in the case of oxygen. Sometimes it takes decades, as in the case of calcium. It's inevitable in any case.

Let's examine oxygen, one of those essential 95 things more deeply. Let's compare its lack with what happens when you take certain drugs.

Suddenly deprive the lungs of oxygen and the effects are fast. Confusion, memory loss, inability to think clearly, all happen immediately, generally quicker than people can think to save themselves.

Inability to focus the mind and the eyes, tunnel vision, blackouts, muscle tremors, weakness and a host of other problems develop in the span of three breaths, the time for oxygen-depleted blood to travel from the lungs to the brain.

They progress to unconsciousness and death in minutes.

However, a feeling of euphoria accompanies the initial symptoms of oxygen starvation.

Does that or does it not sound like the symptoms caused by potent painkillers?

The immediate cure for oxygen deficiency is obvious. Provide oxygen. In the case of painkillers, there is no immediate cure. The kidneys and liver primarily must filter or metabolize these agents out of the blood stream and somehow eliminate them from the body.

Oxygen is only one nutrient. We have to have it continuously because there is so much of it around us and the body doesn't have to store very much internally. Similarly, a person perishes of thirst in a matter of days. A fish, which lives in water, will die quickly when taken out of water.

We need three classes of foods: proteins, carbohydrates and fats. We can live without food for around 6 weeks, sometimes longer, as Gandhi repeatedly showed. You know all of that.

THE NUTRITION REVOLUTION

This book is more about failing to provide food nutrition than air or water. However, the ill effects of air and water deprivation are easier to demonstrate. They are immediate.

The visible effects of food starvation are caused by the body depleting its internal stores of food. It literally stays alive by feeding on itself. For instance, muscles shrivel to provide nutrition for the heart, brain and other more vital organs.

The story continues with another 90 Essential Nutrients for our body. They are less plentiful than protein, carbohydrates and fats, although do we get them from food. Since they are less plentiful, we store more. Because we store more, we can skip days, months, even years. We can live for years without replenishing some of these 90, but without them, disease is inevitable.

When the farmland is depleted of these Essential Nutrients, as it usually is, so is our food from plants and our food from the animals that eat plants, etc. The food chain begins with plants. When the land is depleted, we must somehow supplement our diets with what is missing.

Most of us are smart enough to provide ourselves with air, water and three kinds of food. That accounts for five. Most of us don't know enough about the other 90. This is exactly why I write. We need all of the essentials. That's why they are called essential.

MODULE 4

Length of Life

Let's return to Doctors' Longevity.

Doctors die at an average age of 57.

The average American lives past age 78. The latest number is 79.5.

So on the average, doctors die Two Decades early.

They must be doing something very wrong. Why is that? It's an important question, well worth examining. After all:

- If, for example, people in Hinkley, California were found to be dying ONE decade before their time, all kinds of scientists should be examining that town's ground, its air, its well water, the power lines, local radioactivity, the electromagnetic spectrum, anything to find an explanation.

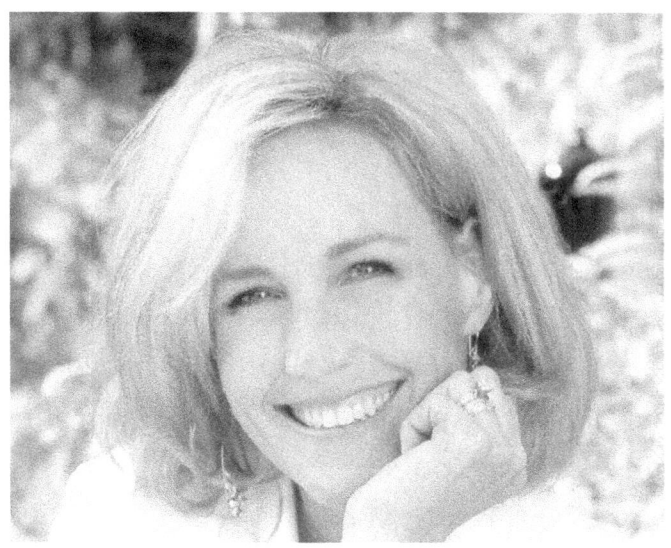

- Remember Erin Brokovich? Despite severe persecution and threats, she found such a culprit. It was hexavalent chromium, aka CR-6 in the industrially poisoned ground water of Hinkley, California, two hours north of where I live. The Pacific Gas and Electric utility company conspired with health officials to conceal the short life spans in Hinkley, so scientists would not wonder why.

Amazingly, the deception continues. A study, released in 2010 by the California Cancer Registry, showed that cancer rates in Hinkley *"remained unremarkable from 1988 to 2008"*. An epidemiologist involved in the study said that the

196 cases of cancer reported during the most recent survey of 1996 through 2008 were less than what he would expect based on demographics and the regional rate of cancer.

Who believes that!

Erin's main contribution was exposing the early deaths caused by terrible forms of cancer, as well as identifying hexavalent chromium in ground water and tracing it to its source, a PG&E plant that used it as an anti-corrosive.

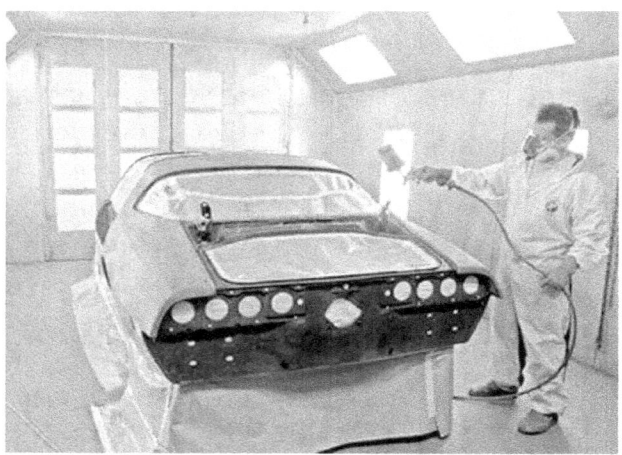

- If a whole profession, such as automotive painters were dying that early all across the nation, there would be an investigation of their work conditions, their materials, anything surrounding their profession. Agencies would spring into action to regulate whatever was causing the problem. There would be fights and lawsuits about who was right about the cause. Headlines would scream.

That actually happened and now some kinds of paint are banned. Other kinds of paint require extreme respiratory gear.

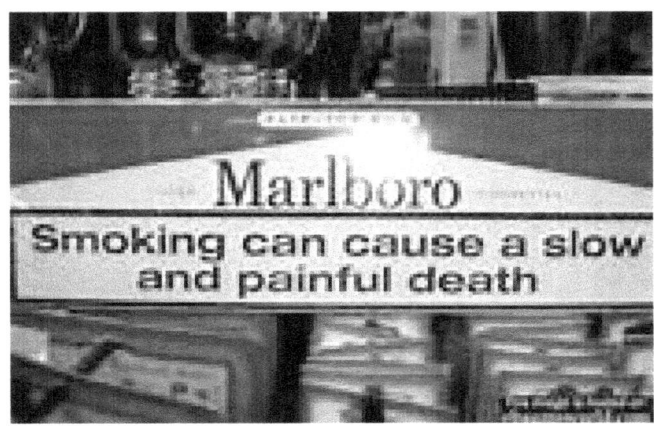

- If a group of people who consumed large quantities of, say, alcohol or cigarettes or lead or mercury, were found to be dying early, governmental agencies would impose stringent notices, safeguards, rules, regulations and laws. Eventually.

This would happen soon after the suppliers of these poisonous products no longer were able to suppress the early death statistics.

THE NUTRITION REVOLUTION

That is precisely what happened to the alcohol, tobacco, paint, asbestos, coal mining and fish industries. First there was denial and suppression. When that tactic failed, the government regulated those industries.

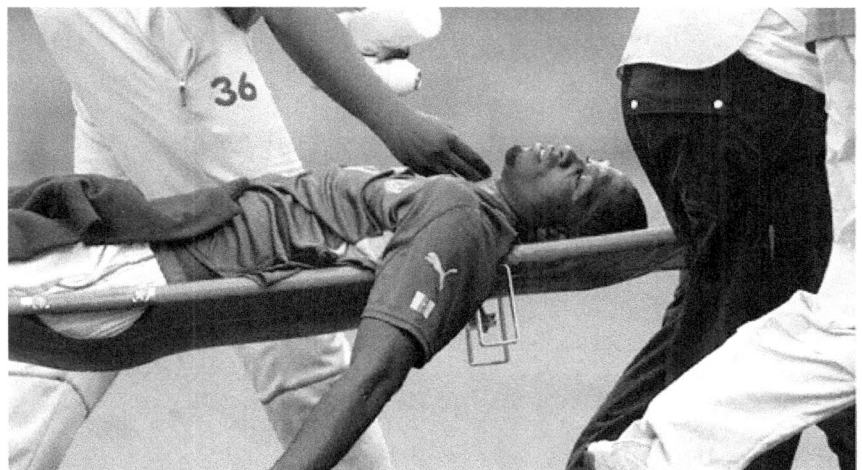

Cardiomyopathy Shocker on the Field of Play.

Why An Average Age Of 57

It's a well-documented fact that physicians die too early. It's revealed in their own records and obituaries. Therefore, it's worth examining the problems that afflict them.

We need our doctors and we need for them to be healthy. We need for them to outlive the rest of us, as examples to follow.

Doctors and the American Medical Association (AMA) have denied and tried to hide the evidence. They are embarrassed over that fact, which tends to indicate that doctors don't understand what they are advising.

The record is clear. Doctors die early at age 57 on the average. Dead Doctors Don't Lie.

One would certainly think that doctors would live longer than the average person, for many reasons:

- They follow their own medical advice.
- They have superb incomes.
- They can afford the most expensive health care.
- They know what that care is, so they can prescribe to their patients.

- They can prescribe to themselves and treat themselves.
- Their colleagues will often provide the finest, cutting-edge care – free.
- They can afford the best food.
- They can afford the newest and best medicines.
- They have a very low-risk profession.
    - About the only risk is catching something from a patient.
    - If they do catch something, they should be able to treat it in themselves as they do with patients. After all, that's why the patient came to them.
- They understand disease prevention.
    - They know how to avoid catching something from a patient. They can take preventative measures on themselves and their families.
- Their suicide rate is low.
- Their car accident rate is low.
- They have wide enforcement powers.

So what is lacking? Why do the physicians die young? Why do they deny the facts?

One common denominator is that they know too little about nutrition and so they neglect it – in their patients and in their own lives.

THE NUTRITION REVOLUTION

A second common denominator is that their profession, their allopathic philosophy, their schooling and most importantly, their suppliers of medicine and equipment conspire against them and keep them in the dark.

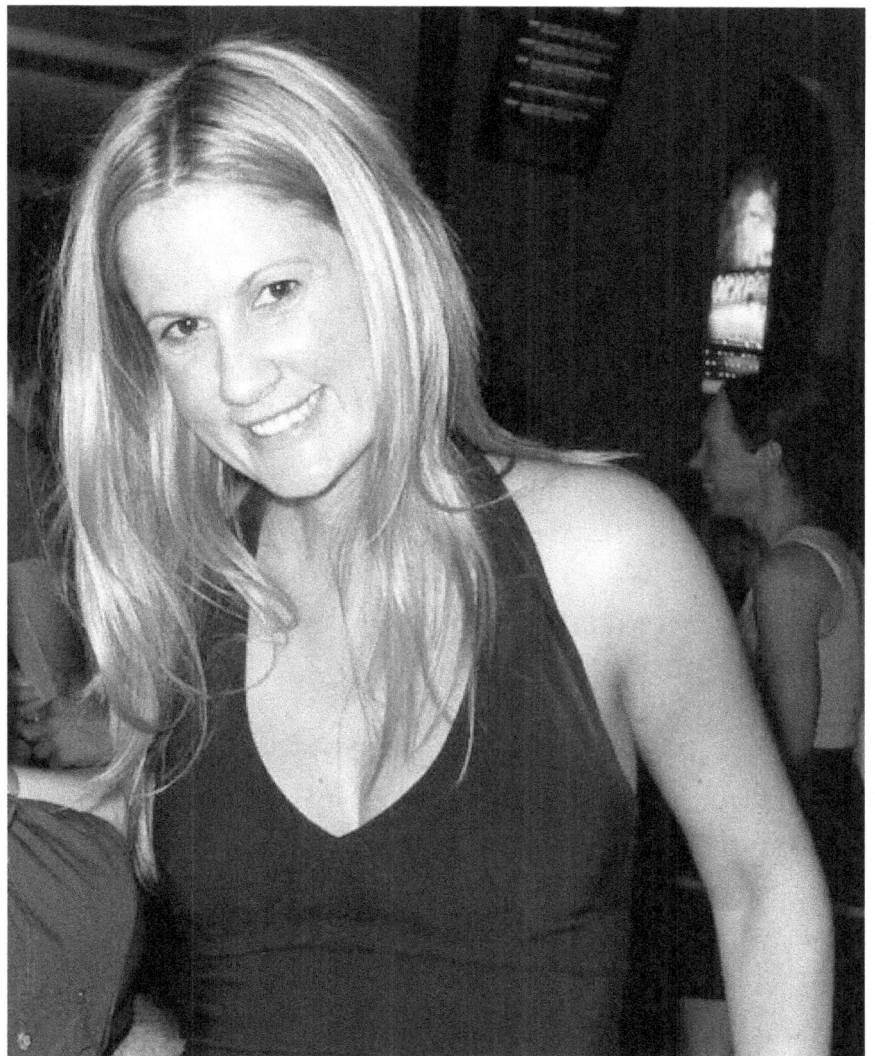

Karni Liddell, Paralympic athlete

MODULE 5

The Role of Big Pharma

It's profitable, highly profitable for medical suppliers to keep physicians in the dark about treatments that would <u>negate the need</u> for mega-dollar scanners, million-dollar regimens of prescription drugs, hugely profitable tests paid for by insurance, etc.

> *I wrote about that profit motive in a thriller novel entitled. "The Seduction of DoctoRx", 2012.*

But wait. So what? Insurance-reimbursed tests are free to the patient, right?

Hardly. Nothing is free. We collectively pay for those tests. Consider insurance premiums to be a tax on the general public, except that it's paid to the insurance companies, instead of to the IRS. Functionally, it's the same thing.

The US Government (Obamacare) even supports this tax. It exceeds income tax for some people.

Do you like your forever-increasing insurance premiums? Do you have any friends who do?

Do you understand why insurance costs have to be so high? The preceding paragraphs and a small amount of thought explain it.

It's a shocker: keeping people sick would be highly profitable, whereas healing them would stop the money stream.

Are all physicians such crass schemers? Of course not! Are some of the leaders in Big Pharma? The evidence and logic are conclusive. Yes, they are.

Deficient Nutrition

Poor nutrition kills people. That's obvious. It kills physicians more quickly than the rest of us, simply because doctors don't know what good nutrition is. Therefore, doctors eat more poorly than the rest of us.

As I wrote, the proof of that disturbing statement is in physician obituaries.

The terrible conclusion is that while we need and honor doctors to let them sew us up on the battlefield and after motorcycle accidents, we can't afford to follow their advice about nutrition.

We would die early, just like they do.

The dead doctors have died young because while they are alive, they were ignorant (or even lied) about nutrition.

I contend that most physicians are highly honorable and high minded. They rarely lie but because they are misinformed by their profession, the effect has been worse. By thrusting themselves into a position of authority and then teaching people error, the effect has been worse than if someone with no reputation taught the same things.

Believing a lie does not make it truth, any more than denying the truth makes it a lie.

Doctors have a moral responsibility to be correct or to say nothing and in my experience most of them do violate that responsibility. When they don't know everything, they should simply say so. Instead, most of them are blindly parroting much of what the large pharmaceutical companies and their universities (who are largely controlled by pharmaceutical companies) and their research papers (largely controlled and sponsored by the same companies) say.

To be fair, most doctors don't like Big Pharma any more than you do.

However, doctors don't have much of a chance. They typically take a single half-hour course in nutrition during their 12 years of college work. Even that course is heavily biased toward eating grains. They simply don't understand nutrition. A slowly-increasing few do, because they've made extraordinary efforts to learn about it, risking their careers, but most don't. Otherwise, they'd protect their lives with great nutrition. They can afford the best.

THE NUTRITION REVOLUTION

A nutritionist can read physician obituaries and recognize nutrition-related diseases that kill doctors early in life. The most common are deficiencies in calcium, copper, selenium and magnesium. How sad!

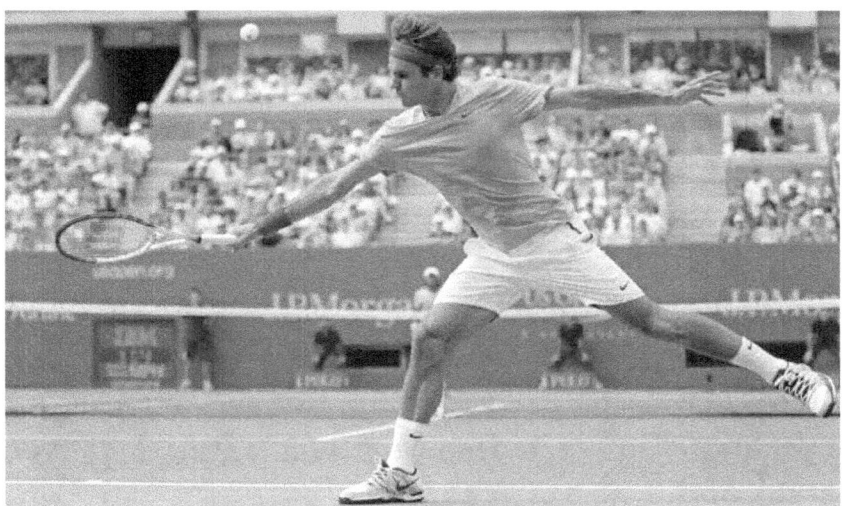

Roger Federer, Tennis Champion,
Poetry in Motion.

MODULE 6

Longevity Limits

Okay, so doctors die at an average age of 57.

Professional athletes don't fare much better at 60. Some, like the Canadian Football League players average about 52.

Nor do billionaires live longer.

The average 'couch potato' who seldom exercises and eats all the wrong foods does a lot better. Couch Potatoes live to around 79.5, (in the USA in 2014) but could live longer. I'll show you how.

It's mathematically trivial to demonstrate that humans have the genetic potential to live far beyond the age of 100. It's a matter of logic and history. If anyone has ever lived past the age of 100, then obviously it's possible!

Has that ever happened? Of course it has.

If someone died at age 110, that means humans have the genetic potential to live at least that long. If someone, anyone, has ever lived past 120, then the potential is at least 120. That's trivial logic.

What is the true potential, even discounting a host of ancients like Methuselah who personally lived to age 969?

There are entire groups of modern people whose elders routinely live past 100, past 110.

> *Jeanne Louise Calment of France, was born February 21, 1837 and lived 122 ½ years. She remains the eldest <u>fully documented</u> human.*
>
> *Source: Wikipedia.*
>
> *There are wide reports, perhaps officially unverifiable because of historical records, of people living 140, 150 and even 170+ years.*
>
> *Hanuman Das Baba is still living. He doesn't know when he was born. However, this Krishna saint's mother was a servant of the Queen of Jhansi, who died in 1858. He was 12 when Jhansi Rani fought the British in 1857. That makes him around 170. The evidence is solid but there is no birth certificate. Those came into being much later.*
>
> *Source: IndiaDivine.org.*

Obviously we have the genetic potential to live past 120, because it has been done.

Interestingly, such long-lived people usually reside far from physicians and have no way to receive doctor care. The reverse is true as well. People in the United States have the finest and most expensive health care in the world. Nobody denies that ...

... except those who look at the results.

Americans spend more on health care than the entire rest of the world, combined. However, we are dead last in infant mortality. We rank 42nd in life expectancy.

We're slipping. It was not always that way. When I was born in 1940, we were first in life expectancy and I remember as a young child hearing we had slipped, not to second, but to fourth in the world that year.

My youthful pride in America took a severe wound that day.

Decades ago, the President of the USA declared war on cancer. It hasn't worked, except that not long ago, Doctors Wallach and Schrauser sued the FDA, spending millions of personal dollars and years of time, proving the efficacy of selenium against several of the worst cancers.

Those doctors forced an inroad on cancer via selenium. They won the lawsuit and now nutritionists or anybody can state that selenium has a positive effect against cancer of the prostate, lungs and breast.

How amazing it is that our honored Food and Drug Administration had to have it proven to them 22 different ways **in front of a judge**, while the FDA spent millions of our dollars defending against a lawsuit!

How amazing it is that they didn't just look at the compelling research a decade earlier and proclaim the selenium results to the world! How amazing it is that they would act on spurious research regarding salt, eggs, cholesterol, etc., that was later proven to be in error. It's as if they have abandoned their solemn duty.

The board of the FDA and the boards of Big Pharma swap members back and forth. Members of the FDA board have heavy, personal investments in various pharmaceutical companies.

Doctor Wallach has sued the FDA seven more times since then and has never lost. One by one, he is proving to the courts and the world that the FDA is suppressing valid treatments.

He, Dr. Glidden and others boldly state that physicians who refuse to treat patients properly, when proper treatment is available, deserve jail time. They say that if a few such MDs did go to jail, the rest would think twice before refusing valid treatment.

However, **if the FDA's main motive is profit**, and if it's hugely profitable to keep people unhealthy, then this situation may not be so amazing after all.

A few forward-looking physicians are beginning to recognize that their profession has been wrong and selenium is important in the fight against cancer. I know two, besides Wallach, Ma Lan and Glidden.

Some are starting to prescribe it.

Selenium <u>alone</u> is not the answer. It is provably effective but it only one of 90 essentials (besides air, food and water.) It needs to be accompanied by the other 89 essential minerals, vitamins, amino acids and fatty acids, plus heavy doses of anti-oxidants so it can be more effective against cancer.

That's the answer; add all of the other essentials. Then selenium is very effective, especially in the presence of ORAC values in the 30,000 range.

> *I consume around 40,000 ORAC points a day. The longest lived people on earth exceed 15,000 a day.*

If you're interested in how effective selenium plus its cofactors can be, please write me for some amazing cases, which many physicians would claim are only spontaneous and temporary remission.

Humph. If cancer is gone, it's gone. Everyone knows that!

If it doesn't return, it doesn't return. That's obvious.

Evidently the FDA doesn't know that because they actually got it into law that it is illegal for <u>anyone</u> to state that such a patient is cured. Physicians who state they cure anyone of anything are breaking the law, thus they never say they cure anything. The only legal thing left for anyone to do is to state that it appears to be gone and it has not returned, yet.

It's interesting that people can shout all manner of offensive obscenities on public TV without breaking the law but if anyone, physicians included, says "selenium has cured some cancers," the law is broken. Physicians can lose their licenses, their jobs and their ability to practice anywhere in the USA.

So if curing disease has been made illegal, I wonder **why, are we still seeking a cure for Cancer?** Or Diabetes? Or Alzheimer's disease? Or Arthritis? Or ADD/ADHD? Or any number of other diseases, which commonly disappear when patients start taking the best nutrition on the planet?

NUTRITION REVOLUTION

A week ago, I heard the story of a lady who had been the top instructor at one of the world's largest medical systems, who reportedly said there are two diseases which will never be cured, simply because there is so much money in them: cancer and diabetes. I suppose I could verify that story if necessary. At this point, it's a third party story.

Earlier, I heard my friend, a prominent California physician state in public that if everyone in California took the Healthy Blood Sugar Pack he designed, there would be no diabetes in California in six months. It's only nutrition. Notably, he didn't bother to mention the connection with sugar. Perhaps it was an oversight. I think it was significant because he is very careful.

Politically, it's a good idea to **try** to cure disease. It wins political points because people want cures.

Financially, it's another story.

This is not a matter of semantics. It's a serious problem.

For one thing, the search for a cure brings in trillions of dollars, whereas finding that cure would stop the huge inflow of research money. Powerful and influential people might have to sell their mansions and jet planes.

Who pays for the search? Why the uncured do, of course. Since nobody is cured of anything, that's everyone.

Is it really that callous?

Ask Jerry Lewis. Okay, his contract says he can't talk. So Google him. His name is enough. I posted an authoritative link on **http://Mktg.Org** about Jerry and "Jerry's Kids." He's the good guy in that story. He's my hero.

Dr. Joel Wallach found the cure and proved it. He could have made a bazillion dollars but he gave it away. He called Jerry. Jerry got excited. He presented it to his sponsors. They fired him.

They even cited a provision in his contract saying he could never talk about the cure or the reason he was fired.

The ex-sponsors **still** rake in billions because we're **still** searching for the cure for Jerry's Kids.

They put Bernie Madoff in jail for less. He stole from rich people like Jerry's ex-sponsors. He didn't go around wasting the lives of children for money.

As Dr. Peter Glidden and others declare widely, *"Someone needs to go to jail!"*

Alzheimer's Disease

I wonder why the spread of Alzheimer's parallels the medical profession's 39 year recommendations of lowered cholesterol levels in the blood.

Three prominent physician friends of mine bluntly call Alzheimer's Disease a "Physician Caused Disease." They cite overwhelming evidence to support that fact.

Alzheimer's Disease appeared out of thin air in the late 1950s, about five years after the medical profession began recommending that people reduce cholesterol in their diets.

I witnessed those two events.

Alzheimer's' spread has paralleled the lowering of cholesterol ever since. That indicates strongly that lowering cholesterol causes Alzheimer's Disease.

I'm a certified master mathematician. I know that when two things are this closely tied, the chances are high that either one causes the other, or else both have the same cause.

> *Furthermore, when there is a sequence, the one that appeared second is probably dependent on the one that appeared first.*

That's very close to being an axiom.

So it appears that Alzheimer's is caused by lowering cholesterol.

In another powerful indicator, people who are not concerned about cholesterol, such as Alaskan Eskimos and Aleuts, don't even have a word for Alzheimer's Disease in their languages. They don't get the disease, despite eating almost nothing but foods high in cholesterol. Since they don't get it, there's no need even to have a word for it.

However, when they abandon their traditional diet and start lowering their cholesterol, they get the same incidences of Alzheimer's Disease and other neurological diseases as everyone else. Those who stay pure to the Eskimo and Aleut diets – don't get the disease.

So it appears that lowering cholesterol probably causes diseases like Alzheimer's, MS, MD, Lou Gehrig's and a host of other neurological diseases. The most respected researchers on earth say certainly, not just "probably."

NUTRITION REVOLUTION

That makes sense when you notice that the brain is 75-80% cholesterol (by weight) and the nerves are about 85% cholesterol. The cholesterol forms the myelin, which is the insulation around every nerve, making sure the nervous signals keep in the correct nerves and go where the body intends them.

Without sufficient cholesterol, the body can't make enough myelin. When that happens, nerves short-circuit, especially in the brain. Signals get misdirected, misguided.

A misguided nervous system means there will be memory loss, twitching, muscular weakness, dizziness, epileptic attacks, seizures. If your brain tells your heart to beat and something else happens instead. That's very bad. Your brain has to tell your heart again and again and your heart skips a beat. Or two. Or more.

If you want your arm to move and instead you kick your spouse at night, I would suspect a lack of cholesterol, instead of that bogus RLS, or Restless Leg Syndrome. TV used to advertise drugs for that. What side effects they had to declare!

Eggs and red meat, which are excellent sources of cholesterol, are still spurned or restricted by most people, because of a couple of spurious scientific studies.

In these specious studies, the evidence seems tainted and even the conclusions are illogical. They use circular reasoning, which magically looks reasonable but proves nothing.

Interestingly, those studies were funded and sponsored by several special interest groups, which would profit by lowered egg and red meat consumption, and others which profit from selling cholesterol-lower drugs. By following the money, you often find the motive.

I want my cholesterol high. I want to remain able to think on my 120th birthday.

Some of the smartest people that I know eat 6 to 10 eggs per day. So do I. Horrors!

I eat plenty of red meat as well as the eggs. I don't want Alzheimer's. At age 80, I can still think as well as ever, writing 12 books in 12 months recently, and two in ten days. I'm running a chain of top-quality vitamin stores, am Dean of a college, am a Trustee of a multi-million dollar enterprise and still find plenty of time to be with my cherished family. It's not me; it's the cholesterol. And the minerals. And the vitamins. Tests show no clogging of my arteries.

Flawed reasoning says that high cholesterol leads to clogging of the arteries. Here's what happens. When arteries clog, the clogging material is mostly cholesterol. The reasoning says that we should reduce blood (serum) cholesterol to prevent these clogs from forming.

The real story, however, is that when the interior artery walls are inflamed, the body uses what flows past, cholesterol, to fight the inflammation. It's rather like forming a scab over a wound, although the process and materials are different. Scabs are made from fibrin, not cholesterol.

The problem isn't the cholesterol, any more than the problem of a wound is the scab.

If a wound develops a staph infection, MRSA or gangrene and you cover it with a bandage so you can't see it, and if you take pills to stop the pain, you will lose the limb or die.

Similarly, if someone interferes with cholesterol levels instead of eliminating the inflammation that causes elevated cholesterol levels, they are covering the real illness.

High cholesterol levels are not dangerous. They are indications, symptoms of a different, potentially dangerous condition, a condition that cries out to be fixed. That condition is inflamed artery walls.

The inflammation is your body telling you that you are deficient in minerals, not that you have too much cholesterol in your blood!

<u>If you're on cholesterol lowering medications, you've got to get out of that trap. You must.</u>

<u>The only way to spring the trap is through proper nutrition and eating enough cholesterol to keep your brain alive.</u>

In February 2015, national news reported that the government is being forced to reverse their warning about cholesterol. The extensive meetings, held in December, 2014 were recorded and put on the Internet. When the members got to cholesterol, one panelist, appeared to bridle, finally stating: <u>"So we're not making a (cholesterol) recommendation. Bummer."</u>

Would you care to check the panelist's investment portfolio? Do you think statins like hugely popular Lipitor or Crestor might be part of it? I didn't check. The proceedings are all recorded on the Internet.

Digestive Diseases

Celiac Disease appeared in massive numbers right after genetically modified (GMO) corn, wheat, barley, rye and oats appeared. These cereals were invented to out-produce older strains of grain and allow saturation-use of pesticides.

As a side-effect, GMO foods contain substantially higher levels of pesticides.

A profitable side effect for companies like Monsanto is that the seeds will grow but their offspring will not germinate. Thus, the farmer is forced to buy new seed each year – from Monsanto et al.

Coincidence? I think it's the law of cause and effect.

Celiac Disease *(aka Coeliac, nontropic sprue, endemic sprue and gluten enteropathy)* is a progressive, nasty, debilitating thing. Sometimes it's called Irritable Bowel Syndrome (IBS.)

As opposed to Alzheimer's, it is an ancient disease identified as early as the 1800s. It affects from 1% to 3% of the population but its spread is increasing.

It destroys the villi lining in the intestines. They are what dissolve nutrients passing through. Without them, the body simply starves. As it progresses, digestion ability diminishes. Along with that, bodies lose the ability to absorb minerals and vitamins, amino acids and essential fatty acids.

Source: Wikipedia and others

So the bodies progressively become more deficient in life-sustaining nutrition. The first treatment that must happen, is to rid the diet of gluten. This means no wheat, barley, rye or oats, at all, forever.

> *Incidentally, there is a wheat allergy, which is entirely different.*

Celiac is a nutrition problem made worse by antacids, which restrict the acid in the stomach needed for digestion.

When my digestion seems less than optimal, I find a glass of orange or grapefruit juice settles things fast! What those acidic beverages do is to raise my stomach's acidity level, not lower it.

Note, however, that grapefruit interferes with the action of about 80 prescription drugs, which I don't want to take anyhow.

NUTRITION REVOLUTION

Digestion requires a high level of acidity. Antacids and acid reducing pills reduce acid. That's the wrong approach.

Harmful organisms in the stomach and intestines die when stomach acid is too high for them. Hooray!

Beneficial organisms flourish. Excellent!

Celiac disease has been linked to IgA deficiency, Dermatitus Herpetiformus, Growth failure, Delayed puberty, Underactive Spleen, hard-to-control Infections, autoimmune disorders, Type-1 Diabetes, Hypothyroidism, Primary Biliary Cirrhosis, Colitis (microscopic) and a number of Pregnancy complications.

It's not yet clear, but several diseases like ataxia, neuropathy, autism and schizophrenia may be linked to Celiac.

A 2015 study links the incidence of type-2 diabetes to GMO foods. That study predicts that in only 20 years, 50% of the USA will have diabetes. Sixty years ago, diabetes was rare.

People with digestive disorders need to avoid gluten (wheat, barley, rye, oats) entirely and forever. They are probably deficient in Calcium, Iron, Folic Acid, Vitamin B12, Vitamin D, Selenium, Copper, Zink and Vitamin K, so supplementation of these nutrients should be increased.

A good food supplement containing extra digestive enzymes and beneficial flora, will aid digestion. It may take a long time to reverse these kinds of diseases but going gluten-free will help quite soon. Minerals and vitamins of the highest absorption and quality will help build the body's strength so it can fight the disease.

The body basically renews itself every few months as cells die and reproduce. Given the correct raw materials, the body's DNA will try with all of its resources (raw materials) to repair the damage.

Cultures and nations, such as most of Europe, which have zero or little celiac disease, coincidentally ban GMO grains – and even the companies like Monsanto, which sell them.

We, also, should rid our diets of GMO foods. Today, it's nearly impossible to stay away from GMO food. Some claim that nearly all people have some degree of Celiac Disease, although it's under different names and in smaller degrees.

Salt and Digestion

I already wrote that salt does not cause or even increase high blood pressure.

The myth that it does was totally discredited years ago. It persists though. A few months ago, I overheard a physician telling a patient to remember to restrict salt in his diet, so he didn't get high blood pressure. I wanted to email him a dozen or so studies but I realized it would be a wasted effort. He's king and I'm not.

"Oh, I will," his patient said, dutifully.

I didn't mention, writing earlier, that salt is necessary for digestion.

The problem with salt reduction is that salt is vital for the production of stomach acid, thus for digestion. Here's how it works:

Table salt is NaCl and stomach acid is HCl. The body merely exchanges Na (sodium) for H (hydrogen) to produce HCl

The body must acquire that NaCl (salt) in the first place. It gets the H from water (H_2O.)

Without good digestion, my ex-doctor's patient will increasingly become deficient in certain minerals that control blood pressure – copper, calcium and magnesium – and will probably develop the life-threatening condition known as high blood pressure.

What was prescribed to lower blood pressure will eventually raise it!

Slightly disgusted, I walked out of the waiting room and canceled my next appointment. When the receptionist called a week later, I told her why I had 'fired my MD.' Her response was to offer to reschedule the appointment, now that I had demonstrated that I knew more than my doctor about salt.

That's great salesmanship!

She also asked that since I have free medical care, why should I care about another patient's health concerns?

Medical care is not free and I do care. Deeply.

I should clarify. As a pilot, I must take annual physical exams or not fly. As a decorated military retiree, I have earned inexpensive (not quite free) medical care, in return for 22 years of service and 106 aerial combat missions. I lost friends. In WW-II, most pilots didn't survive twenty combat flights.

I care enough that I want to go to a physician who doesn't make such blatant mistakes as telling someone to restrict salt to lower blood pressure! Bloodletting will lower blood pressure too. Nobody would recommend that!

I have noticed since childhood that a wound tastes more salty than the surrounding skin. Now I know why. A study done at Vanderbilt University shows that the body accumulates massive amounts of sodium (component of table salt) locally, to boost immune response wherever needed.

That would include such things as artery walls, stomach lining and intestine lining, which become inflamed. Those inflammations contribute to or cause:

- High blood pressure due to clogged arteries and cardiovascular disease,

- Ulcers,

- Celiac and its myriad of cousins.

Rubbing salt into a wound hurts! Now we know why anyone would even consider doing that. Salt has been known for centuries to help cleanse a battle wound and prevent infection. It turns out that the *"Sodium deposits build up where skin infections take place, increasing the activity of immune cells called macrophages that consume microbes."*

Jens Titze, Vanderbilt Universith, Nashville, TN. The study is at http://utsandiego.com/saltinfection

MODULE 7

Financial Aspects

At times, Doctors are wrong in other ways that benefit them and their employers financially. A friend of ours canceled her knee replacement because her knees were doing so much better now that she had corrected her mineral deficiency with nutrition and had added glucosamine and chondroitin to her diet. Her physician agreed with her. Good for him!

Knee replacement surgery starts at around $35,000 per knee and has common complications. Complications cost extra. Much extra.

Some complications threaten lives.

When the same friend called about another condition caused by a calcium and magnesium deficiency, the <u>receptionist</u> tried mightily to reschedule the knee replacement, with a <u>different</u> physician to do the work. This happened at probably the finest hospital in that half of her state.

The **receptionist, who is not a doctor** was clearly practicing medicine without a license by selling, recommending and prescribing a medical procedure. The fact that the new physician would probably ratify the receptionist's recommendation – does not diminish the fact that she was practicing illegally.

The hospital, perhaps not so fine after all, pestered her for three weeks, until our friend told them emphatically *"Put me on your do not call list."*

She no longer has the other condition either. It wasn't legally "cured" of course. Curing is impossible, according to the law, but she no longer has it and is healthier in many other ways. If it's gone, it's gone.

I mentioned deadly side effects. Another dear friend, who'd recently had an optional, double knee replacement, nearly died suddenly. He developed a fast-spreading, excruciating, life-threatening infection in his new knee. He spent a week in the hospital, during which time they opened his knee and cleaned out the infection, barely averting amputation They saved his life. He received much prayer.

There is only one possibility. The infection had to be caused by something not sterile in the operating room, as if any operating room could ever be completely sterile. Industrial clean rooms are more sterile than hospital operating rooms!

> *As evidence, despite Herculean procedures and precautions, professionals who tend to Ebola patients catch and succumb to that disease. Almost nothing can filter out viruses and bacteria – certainly not the masks surgeons and nurses wear to breathe. It is said that Ebola is not airborne.*

After a week, the hospital let our friend go home but required him to return every day for massive doses of intravenous antibiotics, the most powerful known to man. They even installed semi-permanent tubes into his veins for the injections. Now, those tubes are removed and he takes massive amounts of antibiotics orally.

It caused a chain reaction. Those antibiotics quickly ruined his digestion by killing the good bacteria needed for digestion – all because of a botched knee replacement. He has to take doses of digestive bacteria every day now.

The hospital might get a small fine but probably won't. The feds reserve token fines for hospitals that have thousands or even tens of thousands of such errors in a year.

On the other hand, if you botch a left turn in your car and injure a pedestrian who might die, you pay a heavy price. Heavy. You might never get to drive or work again.

Our friend's surgeon has undoubtedly performed knee replacements ever since, at perhaps $35,000 apiece. Like your successful left turns, most of those surgeries probably work out fine.

Highly skilled surgeons and those who police them obviously hold themselves to a <u>lower</u> standard than ordinary drivers making left turns.

MODULE 8

Kinds of Medical Practice

Allopathic Medicine

Doctors are taught to take an 'allopathic' view of the body. This means that they only treat the specific part of the body, which seems to be malfunctioning.

That's fine if the problem is a bullet wound. Doctors are extremely good at fixing things like that. Battlefield medicine is nothing short of amazing.

Medical science's ability to eliminate infection is also strong, despite the fact that several superbugs thwart doctors regularly. If you catch one of these infections, it is almost always going to be in a hospital.

In general, however, a disease does not affect just one body part.

If an elbow has arthritis, the condition exists all through the body.

Even cancer is rarely localized. Some tumors are slow spreading, but they are rarely localized for long.

Diabetes is systemic. It affects the entire body.

Digestion problems are not just in the stomach and intestine because they affect the entire body.

A diseased kidney isn't the only part of the body that's ill. The sickened kidney might be only the symptom of a disease that the kidney is trying to cure by filtering out the toxins the disease is causing.

Alternately, the diseased kidneys might be sick because they've been filtering out prescribed drugs, like statins, which damage kidneys and other organs, attempting to alleviate some other condition.

The allopathic approach isolates things and treats them separately. It's a seemingly logical approach that is wrong in most cases, the exceptions being trauma and certain kinds of localized infections.

Homeopathic Medicine

Nearly all diseases, syndromes, conditions and medical problems are Homeopathic in nature. Homeo indicates all-inclusive. It pertains to the whole body, not just parts.

Another word might be Systemic.

This means that the entire body is sick, not just one part. So the whole body must be treated, not just a single part.

Things like arthritis, diabetes and ADHD are systemic, homeopathic, whole-body illnesses.

In general all chronic illnesses are Systemic. Chronic diseases are those which persist for a long time, even a lifetime – as opposed to Acute diseases like a throat infection that the body is able to cure.

Often a physician prescribes something to assist the body in curing itself. As an example, an antibiotic can help cure an infected wound but even the physician admits that the human body cures itself. The antibiotic merely immobilizes or kills the offending bacteria. The wound caused by the infection remains. The body makes the resulting wound heal.

It takes a homeopathic approach to help the body cure itself. No legal entity can fault the body for curing itself, so the 'cure' word is entirely appropriate.

Dr. Linus Pauling, two-time Nobel Prize winner, stated, "You can trace every disease and ailment to a mineral deficiency."

He went a little further, stating that all diseases go away if treated with proper nutrition.

It takes a homeopathic approach to <u>prevent</u> and to <u>reverse</u> nearly all diseases.

Dr. Pauling's stature trumps the stature of just about any other doctor.

Nutrition is homeopathic. It affects the entire body in a positive way.

The difference between Homeopathic and Allopathic medicine is easily illustrated.

NUTRITION REVOLUTION

Car engines wear out. Mechanics insert new parts or repair worn parts with new materials. Replacing parts is an allopathic approach to a car. A homeopathic approach would be likened more to:

- Filling the gas tank before the engine burns out its catalytic converter by running out of gas.

- Topping off the radiator before the engine overheats and ruins its pistons, rings and cylinders.

- Keeping the oil level correct to preserve various bearings.

- Adding brake fluid to prevent what might in a human be analogous to a sudden catastrophe like a stroke.

Those are systemic or homeopathic actions.

Replacing the brake pads would be more of an allopathic action, akin to repairing a blown-out knee for a football player.

Our bodies wear out too. The good Lord created our bodies to heal themselves. He knew that our bodies would wear out, just like machines that we create.

He made our bodies able to repair themselves, but we mortals have never mastered that trick for things we make. Our creations, machines, cannot repair themselves. When a machine's part wears out, a mechanic rebuilds or replaces it.

Before a body part wears out, the built-in design is for the body to rebuild it, not replace it.

A doctor could **replace** a knee or hip joint. That would be an allopathic action, but **the body can rebuild the hip joint itself,** if given the proper building materials. That's a homeopathic action. The main building materials in this case are:

- Calcium
- Several cofactors of calcium like strontium and magnesium
    - These cofactors facilitate the absorption of calcium by critical cells
- Glucosamine
- Chondroitin
- Gelatin (really!)

The same gelatin you eat for strong, healthy fingernails helps rebuild your joints as they wear.

The body takes these building materials and via amazingly complex internal processes it rebuilds bone and even cartilage. Analogous to blueprints, it uses patterns encoded into its marvelous DNA. The DNA specifies exactly what needs to go where, molecule by molecule. When things are missing, DNA tells the body to scavenge around for what goes there. The body gets the raw materials from its internal storage or from nutrition.

> *The Harvard School of Medicine has a beautiful, must-see animation series showing what happens in a human cell. It is called, "The Inner Life of a Cell." Winkey Pratney showed me it, commenting that there's more going on in one cell than in New York City.*
>
> *Here is a link for you to type into your browser.*
>
> *http://tinyurl.com/kjta77u*

This is only one such video of several. Follow other links. From there, other fascinating videos can be clicked. That cute little guy dragging a huge blob is called a motor protein. He is taking a protein module to the place it goes.

He's going somewhere with a purpose. How does he know where to go? I suspect that if you could ask him, he'd say the Creator tells him, using DNA as the blueprint.

There are millions of motor proteins in every cell. You probably have a million cells in a fingertip. Here's an image from a video shared by Harvard Medical School:

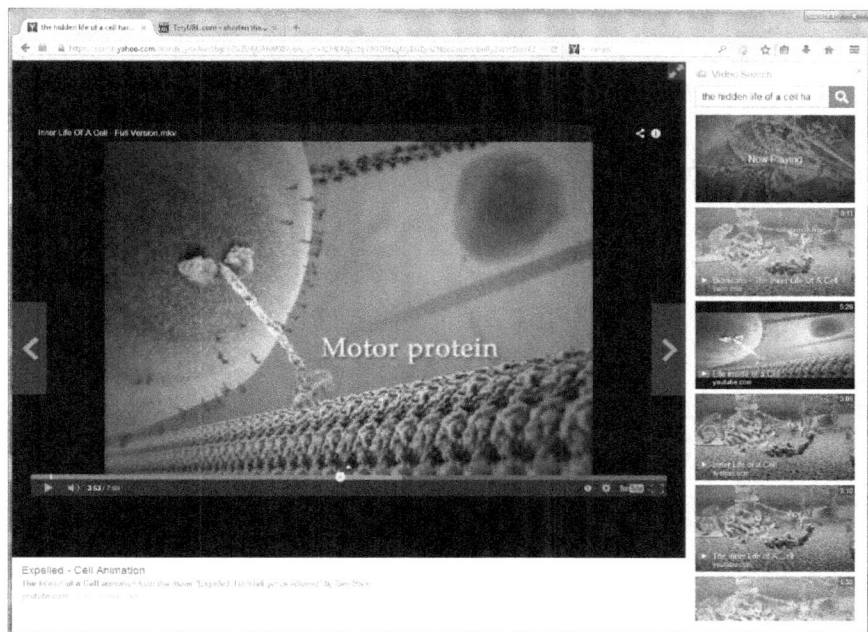

http://tinyurl.com/kjta77u

MODULE 9

How Nutrition Works

Oxygen, water, protein, carbohydrates and fats account for five of the 95 things we need to stay alive: There are 90 left to discuss.

Of those 90, we need 60 essential minerals, 16 vitamins, 12 amino acids and at least 2 fatty acids. They are called "essential" because our bodies cannot manufacture those things. Consumption is essential.

For example: cholesterol is something that our bodies need but **can** manufacture in the liver, although in insufficient quantity.

Cholesterol is not considered an essential element for survival, because our livers can make most of what we need. Even so, if we starve our diets of cholesterol, we will get sick and die of nervous and brain degenerative diseases. We must consume some cholesterol to replace the stores of cholesterol our bodies continually need for scores of mental and nervous repairs.

Calcium is Essential.

We cannot manufacture calcium in our bodies, so it's called "Essential." Nothing short of the sun or original creation can manufacture calcium. (Atomic piles can, at huge cost, millions of dollars for a piece the size of a grain of salt.)

Plants cannot manufacture it, but they can pull it up from the soil, that is, if it is present into the soil. Calcium, in relatively large quantities, is absolutely essential to human life and all animal life.

Even boneless creatures like sharks and jellyfish have cartilage and muscle, which requires calcium for formation and repair.

Calcium is the most abundant mineral in the human body. We find it in bones and teeth, but the body needs it for many other essential activities. A severe calcium deficiency causes 147 different diseases, including the obvious one and its cousins, osteoporosis.

The role of calcium in osteoporosis is logical. When the body is deficient in calcium, it pulls calcium from the bones, making the bones (osteo) porous and brittle.

THE NUTRITION REVOLUTION

Less expectedly, calcium deficiency causes a diverse number of other diseases. The brain and nerves need calcium. Calcium helps regulate the heartbeat. The muscles need calcium, and when they lack calcium, cramps are inevitable.

About muscles: as an aside, I used to fly airplanes for the Air Force and I was as fit as any pilot at age 30. However, unusual exercise would cause me muscle pain the next day sometimes lasting three days. That happens to everyone, right?

That was a long time ago when I had somewhat more stamina and strength than I do now. It was worth my life to be in good shape because in a dog fight, except for surprise and a superior aircraft, the victor is the pilot whose body is best. Aerial combat is as demanding as an Olympic gymnastic floor exercise. In different ways, it requires greater skill and mental ability.

Success is far more obligatory! The victor gets to live, putting a premium on fitness. The defeated only hopes to survive a crash or a punishing ejection seat ride.

This past Good Friday, 2014, I took a group of people to Hilltop Park in San Diego, where there's a huge soccer field. I was showing them how to fly four-line stunt kites, quite an athletic endeavor. I was running all over the field helping this person or that person keep a kite in the air. They were spaced about 200 feet apart, but they were largely stationary. I was running around launching kites.

After about three or four hours of my running around like this, they were asking me to go home. They were tired and they were sure their bodies would be sore the next day. So we went home but the next day we did it again.

I figured that I would be sore the next day but no. I was not. Once again, I ran all over the soccer field for three or four hours showing people how to fly kites. Toward the end, they were dropping like flies, winding up their strings and seeking park benches, while I still ran around showing the remnant how to fly.

The next day, Easter Sunday, I was still not sore and I played the saxophone in church services, like I always do.

I was 73 years old that day. I don't exercise much. If I had tried that at age 30 or 40, unless I had worked up to that level of exercise, I would have been extremely sore for three or four days.

THE NUTRITION REVOLUTION

I was a skier back then and I knew to begin about six weeks before ski season, exercising and practicing the moves in my living room. Even then, after I returned from the mountains, I would be hurting and barely fit to fly for a couple of days.

The reason is that back in those days when I was a fit and healthy pilot, I was not taking enough calcium. Nobody knew. Today I take plenty of calcium, and that was, to me, proof that my body needs calcium to prevent muscle soreness and cramps.

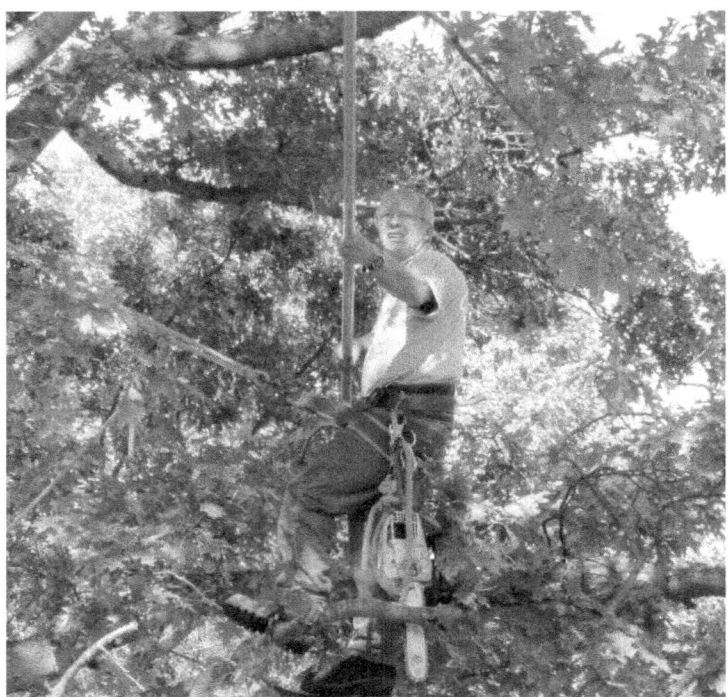

This tree trimmer looks just like my brother John, but he's someone else. Uncanny resemblance.

The fact hit home again today. My nephew, Jason and I spent most of yesterday with a chain saw and hand loppers, lacing and pruning a tree, cutting the branches into two-foot lengths, raking, cleaning out bushes and the like. I haven't done that for thirty years. Today, I have zero muscular soreness. The only thing I feel different is a bit stronger.

As important as calcium is, we have rather significant amount of calcium stored in our bodies, and we can go without it for a lot longer than we can go without food. Calcium is, however, essential to human life, and without it the body will perish.

Role of Magnesium

Magnesium is another mineral to which our bodies have become dependent and accustomed. Magnesium is something we can't make, so it's 'essential.' Magnesium helps the body absorb calcium and has other magnificent benefits. One thing it does is to open certain receptors on cells to allow the calcium to enter and exit. Magnesium is called a co-factor for calcium. There are other co-factors for calcium, such as strontium. You need them all.

Supplementation

One of the lies that dead doctors tell until they die is that ordinary calcium supplementation will do the trick. They presume that most of the ingested calcium is used and not excreted.

The big fat truth is that only calcium that has gone through plants is usable. Calcium from rocks is about 3% absorbable. The rest is excreted as waste. From plants, the absorption rises to more than 97%.

The problem is that the calcium must be in the correct form, or our bodies cannot absorb it. It's a matter of particle size and electrical charge.

As with most of the minerals, calcium supplements usually come from rocks. In the case of calcium the rock is dolomite, which is calcium magnesium carbonate, $CaMg(CO_3)_2$. You find the same material in seashells, coral and the water deposits around your water faucets. Geologically, most dolomite used to be seashells and coral. In one form, over time, it got compressed into the rock dolomite.

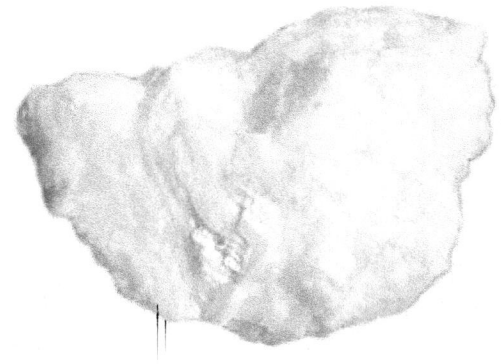

In another form, it got dissolved and redeposited as crystals like these white ones.

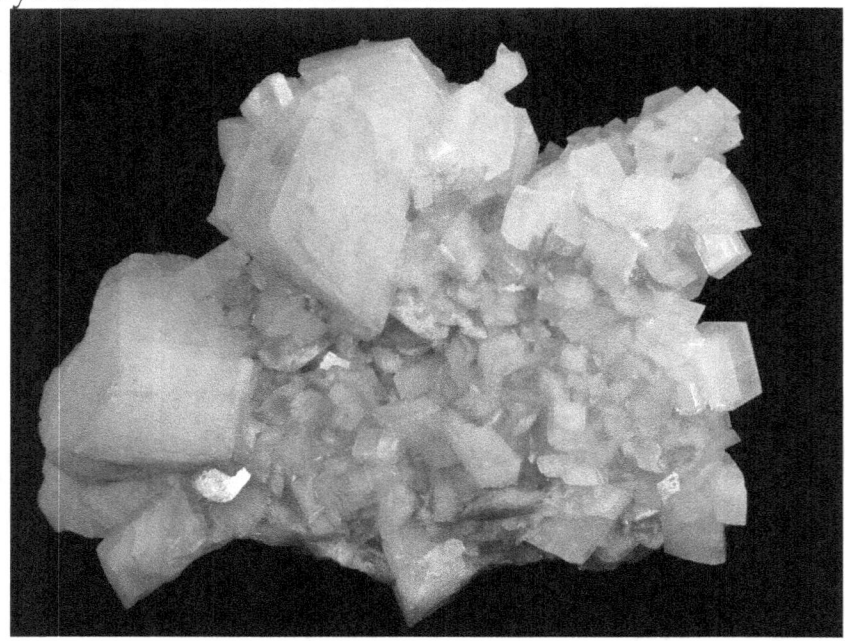

Seashells and coral are mostly calcium magnesium carbonate, along with just a few other minerals. $CaMg(CO_3)_2$ is high in calcium (Ca) and Magnesium (Mg). One would think that we can grind up dolomite into powder and then hard press it into pills for a good source of calcium.

Absorption

The problem with that idea is that the pills are composed of minute granules of rock flour, or seashell flour or coral flour. Each particle is perhaps 1,000 times larger than a human cell, no matter how finely we grind the rocks. Because of that fact, hard pressed calcium pills, which are not very expensive, are only about 2% or 3% absorbable by the body. The rest is wasted.

An ordinary person needs around 1,200 milligrams of calcium every day. A person fighting calcium deficiency needs far more, for a time.

Many calcium pills on the market contain 1,200 mg per pill. If only 3% of the calcium a person takes is absorbable, that means they have to consume about 33 pills per day! If it's 2%, then the math says they need to choke down 50 pills per day.

It gets worse. A body can only process about 500 mg at a time in this form (powdered rock,) so one would need eat those pills, spaced out evenly during the day and night.

That could cause some digestive problems!

The problem is that 3% absorbability.

Solutions

The solution is getting calcium from food. However, it's difficult to get enough calcium from food. Most people in the United States are severely calcium deficient.

I remember loving milk as a kid. My parents said it was high in calcium and made for strong bones. I got plenty, until about age 12 when a pediatrician asked my parents to restrict milk so I'd eat more food and gain weight faster. I now think this milk contributed to my present health.

The problem of insufficient calcium (and other minerals) in our diet has an elegant solution, provided by the earth, itself.

A long time ago, there was a gargantuan volcanic eruption in the state of Utah, covering 200 square miles. Over hundreds of years, a forest naturally grew up on top of that cap rock, as forests do. Their roots reached deep into the rock and extracted at least 71 different minerals, 60 of which are known to be essential to human life. The plants created their own thick, rich topsoil, containing all of those minerals. Then another geologic event placed another cap of rock over the plants, encapsulating and compressing their mineral goodness into a special kind of shale, for us to mine. These <u>plant derived</u> minerals are already in <u>colloidal form</u>, perfect for human consumption. So what are colloids?

Colloids

Plants have the amazing, unmatched ability to make nutrient particles small enough to enter tiny plant cells. In this form, the mineral particles are called colloids. They are about 7,000 times smaller than a human cell, so they can pass into and out of human cells easily. They don't accumulate into toxicity.

In the case of calcium, ground-up rock particles are far larger than human cells. They can't fit in. Being millions of times smaller in comparison, colloidal calcium particles are about 7,000 smaller than human cells. For this reason, colloidal calcium is about 97% to 98% absorbable by the human body, whereas rock-derived calcium is about 3% bioavailable.

A colloid particle might be 1/7,000,000 the size of a grain of rock flour. In that instance a gram of colloidal calcium has almost two-trillion (1,993,815,104) times as much **surface area** as a gram of rock flour! That surface area is part of why colloidal particles enter and exit cell walls so readily.

> *This also explains why a spoonful of sugar dissolves so much faster than an equal amount of rock candy. Dissolving occurs at the surface of each particle. Rock candy has a tiny amount of surface area, compared to granular sugar.*

It's no wonder colloidal calcium is so much more bio-available than ground up rocks.

There's another reason, which is probably more important. <u>Colloidal particles have the opposite electrical charge from cells.</u> Colloids have positive charges.

Rock particles have the same charge as cells. They both have negative charges.

As you know, opposites attract. The same kinds of charges repel each other. So cells actively seek colloids. Just as actively, they repel rock particles. A poor rock can't get an even chance!

A person can get all of his or her calcium requirement out of 2 tablespoons, (one fluid ounce) of liquid, plant-derived, colloidal calcium, as opposed to 33-50 large calcium pills.

The plants in that ancient forest contained, in their tissues, all of the minerals we need for nourishment.

Youngevity has a perpetual and exclusive rights to this encapsulated shale. No one else can get it. It's all on federal park land in the state of Utah. It's nearly unique.

> *To be complete, there is one other such deposit known, a small one in China. Dr. Ma Lan has visited it. Unfortunately, that site's mineral content is too low.*

Effectively, there is only one commercially available source of plant derived colloidal calcium in the world, and only Youngevity can mine it.

Calcium is only one of 60 minerals that are essential to human life, and all 60 are in that shale, in correct proportions.

In summary, colloidal sized minerals are supremely bio-available. Other forms of mineral supplements are simply not bio-available enough. You would have to take far too much, in the form of pills, to get enough.

One fluid ounce (1/4 cup) of colloidal calcium is the equivalent of at least 33 large calcium pills.

Vitamins

As dire as the mineral situation is, the story worsens.

Plants need these minerals to make the vitamins, amino acids and fatty acids that are so essential to human life. Plants grown in mineral-poor soil not only lose taste, they are deficient in vitamins, amino acids and fatty acids. Most commercial farmland soils are depleted of minerals so plants don't taste as good and lose their ability to make these essential nutrients.

> *For example, in year 2000, scores of square miles immediately to the west of our home were devoted to tomato farming, with a few strawberry operations interspersed. Now that land is developed into housing. Recently, we discovered the reason. We had noticed it without knowing why.*

> *For decades, the tomato and strawberry growers tested their soils annually. Nutritional value was dropping. Tomatoes were losing their taste. Strawberries were too. We stopped buying produce from that area because it tasted like water. That's what we'd noticed, without knowing the reasons.*

> *Finally, the land was so depleted that it was only usable for houses, so up sprang the housing developments west of our home.*

THE NUTRITION REVOLUTION

That accounts for vitamin and amino acid content. The story of fatty acids is similar in some ways. Humans can obtain fatty acids from evening primrose oil, but the best source is ocean fish. Most fish live in waters relatively near the continents, where food supplies are best.

Rivers contain silt, which contains minerals. By way of the food chain, fish are dependent on the minerals in silt, to create the fatty acids we need.

Mankind invented hydroelectric dams to generate electricity. These dams stop and store the river water, then release it to turn turbines and produce electricity.

The nutritional problem with dams is that the rivers' silt no longer makes its way to the ocean. It builds up behind the dams, instead of falling out into the ocean to nourish fish. We are losing our oceans. Fish are rare out in the deep blue water. Fish near the coast are deficient in essential fatty acids.

Thus, we must supplement our fatty acids too.

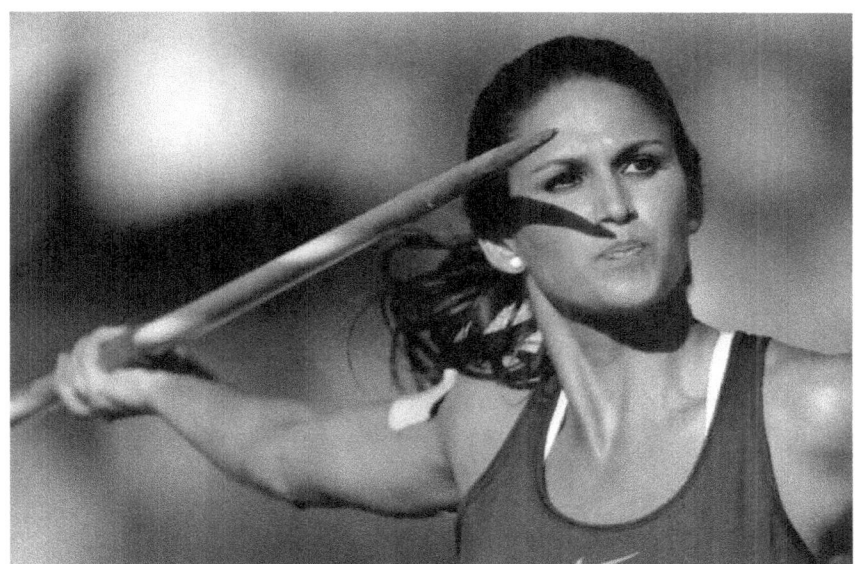

Leryn Franco, Javelin

MODULE 10

Farmland Depletion

A U.S. gov't study, produced in 1937, stated that the farmlands are depleted. That was 1937. Imagine today. In general, towns and cities are sustained by the farmlands within about 100 miles.

Earlier I wrote that when plants have taken all of the minerals out of the soil into their cells, there is no practical mechanism on earth to replace them.

> *Atomic reactors made plutonium for the A-Bomb at a cost of a hundred billion dollars per golf ball sized sphere, half a century ago.*

The point is that what has gone from the soil is gone forever.

Farmers are business people. They must run their farms at a profit, or they will go bankrupt and then there's no farm. Farmers understand that plants grow nice and green and look very healthy, if they are given only three minerals: nitrogen (N), potassium (K) and phosphorus (P). Fertilizer has an NKP rating, which states the percentage of N, K and P in it. 20-20-15 fertilizer has those percentages of minerals and the rest (45%) is inert. That is a strong fertilizer, by the way.

Farmers spread nitrogen, potassium and phosphorus on their fields for increased 'yield' and for plants that look good, long after the soils are depleted of the other minerals. Such good-looking plants don't taste as good and they don't have the vitamins that people crave. Plants grown in those environments where the soil is lacking minerals, are causing people to starve of most of the other minerals we need for life – as well as vitamins, amino acids and fatty acids.

In this case, good looks don't matter.

It doesn't make a lot of sense to ship foods far across the country if they can be locally grown. This means that after 10 or 20 years, when they land around a given city is mostly depleted of essential minerals, the people of that city, any city, are getting minerally deficient food. It also means that they're getting food deficient in vitamins and amino acids because plants need minerals to make those things.

It's the same for small towns.

That's why houses now occupy the former tomato and strawberry fields west of our San Diego home.

To reiterate, our bodies have storehouses of these minerals and vitamins, amino acids and fatty acids, and we can live for a long time with deficiencies in some of them. Eventually, diseases will occur when essentials are missing. When the diseases ravage the body, sometimes the effects are long-lasting or permanent. In other cases the disease can be arrested and reversed by providing the body with the correct items.

Our only recourse is supplementing our diets.

Summary

All Nutrients In Correct Amounts

For any nutrient, there is a minimum amount we need, and a maximum amount we can tolerate. If the nutrients are colloidal minerals, the span between minimum and maximum is quite wide. In metallic form, however, the span can be rather narrow and toxicity is more likely.

Arsenic, studied earlier is such an example. A more common example is iron. We need iron but as pregnant women are taught, we can ingest too much iron too. Each mineral has a proper, therapeutic level for optimum health.

It's the same for just about everything, even things like water and air. We need oxygen, obviously, but it is possible to have too much oxygen. Breathing high pressure, 100% oxygen for extended periods of time causes all sorts of bad things to happen to a body. Oxygen is quite corrosive but the body has elaborate mechanisms for keeping the corrosion, oxidation, in the proper places. Our bodies use oxygen to corrode, that is, break down, hundreds of compounds, turning them into fuel. Too much oxygen, for too long, gets around the body's controls.

Oxygen helps cure some conditions because oxygen is quite toxic to many living things, especially at higher pressures. That's called hyperbaric therapy. It can't be extended indefinitely.

Similarly we need water but if we drink too much water, the body can't stand it and we get sick. If the water gets in the wrong places, such as the lungs, we drown and that's not even what I'm writing about. People who drink too much water get sick from water poisoning. We need to drink the correct amount of fluid every day.

THE NUTRITION REVOLUTION

What all of this means is, for anything our body needs, there is a minimum amount and there's a maximum amount. We must have at least the minimum and we should not have more than the maximum.

It's the same for each of these:

- All 60 minerals,
- All 16 vitamins
- All 12 amino acids
- Both fatty acids
- Air
- Water
- Protein
- Carbohydrates and
- Fat.

We need each one of those nutrients and we need them of the proper amount, not too much and not too little.

Colloids

Over time, our bodies have learned to expect the 60 essential minerals, in the same ratios found in the semi-shale that Youngevity mines in Utah. Moreover, those minerals are colloidal in form. Their particles are exactly the proper sizes and carry the proper charges to enter into our cells, and to exit if cells have too much of them.

Shales

These shales have exactly what our bodies have grown to expect.

Notice that these shales are not from depleted farmland!

> *Youngevity calculated that there is enough humic shale in their Utah mining operation to supplement the entire world's food supply for at least 200 more years.*

THE NUTRITION REVOLUTION

Depletion

Animals and fish live on plants or on other animals that eventually live on plants. Plants are at the bottom of the food chain. If their environments are depleted of minerals, even the meat is low in the proteins, fats, amino acids and fatty acids we need.

Physician Understanding

Unfortunately, medical doctors almost universally do not understand this process. It's hardly their fault; they simply have almost no training in it. Moreover they are allopathic physicians, who are trained to treat specific pieces of the body, not the whole body at a time.

Supplementation

There is only one inexpensive answer to our dilemma. We have to supplement our diets with the 90 Essential minerals, vitamins and fatty acids.

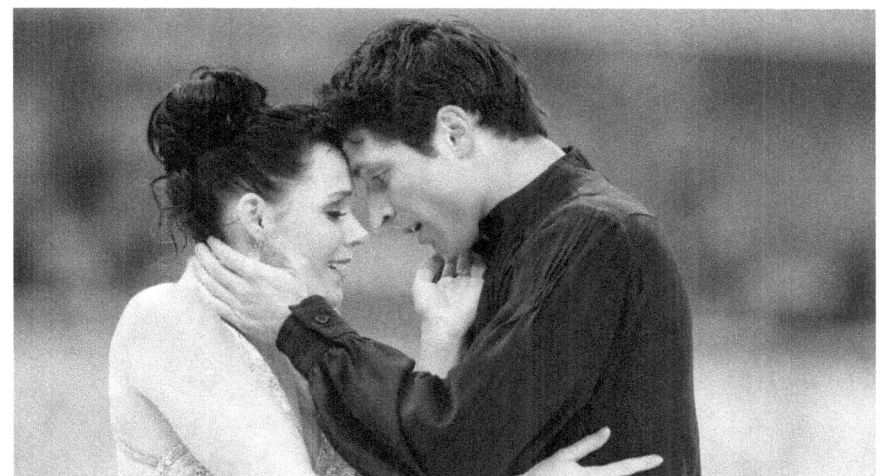

Tessa Virtue and Scott Moir, Canadian Gold
Medalists in Ice Dancing.

MODULE 11

The Problem of Big Pharma

There are many things wrong with the large pharmaceutical companies and the FDA.

Alopathy

For one thing, they are training physicians to promote and prescribe drugs to treat specific part of the body, not the whole body. That's allopathic medicine.

Advertising

For another, they lobbied successfully for the right to advertise directly to consumers instead of just to doctors. Their profits vaulted.

TV is about 50% commercial time these days. A typical three-minute commercial for a prescription drug, is filled with images of people having a grand time, playfully enjoying a tire swing or jogging on the beach. The narrator spends 2-1/2 minutes reciting the mandatory list of terrible things that can happen to you if you take this drug – and then has the temerity to say, *"Ask your doctor if <that drug> is right for you."*

Well, duh!

One of the currently advertised drugs, an anti-depressant, actually says that if you have increased depression or thoughts of suicide after taking it, you should stop taking it.

That makes sense!

It shouldn't be on the market!

It makes better sense not to take it in the first time because it causes depression and it's billed as an anti-depressant.

Outside-The-Laboratory Drug Testing

Large pharmaceutical companies don't just encourage doctors to prescribe their medicines. They pass out billions of dollars' worth of free samples to try on patients. A Physician's Assistant once told my wife, *"This drug is pricey but I have free samples. Let's see if it works."*

A highly respected physician told my wife and me last year, *"The average drug only works on 50% of the patients. The very best work about 70% of the time."*

In other words, let's try this and see what happens. If not, or if you have a dangerous reaction, let's try something else.

This turns the patients into Guinea pigs, in many cases, because the doctors are sincerely interested in finding out if the drug will help the patient.

Lab testing is hugely expensive because of enormous risks. Testing by physicians on patients is almost free because patients take the risks.

Because no drug company can stand the bad press of killing babies, (remember Thalidomide?) drugs are almost never tested on children under five years of age. There are a few exceptions. Instead, physicians do the testing "off label" and if the child's health suffers, well the drug companies are off the hook. They aren't responsible.

Pushing Drugs

I wrote a book called, "The Seduction of DoctoRx." It's a chiller and thriller of a novel, but it is also an expose' of some of the worst practices by big pharmaceutical companies.

The Seduction of DoctoRx begins with the deaths of several children due to off-label prescriptions – all hushed up of course, but the Governor of California happens to be one of the parents.

What follows, the investigations, the cover-ups, the findings, the salesmanship, the intrigue, the conspiracy, the murders, the frame-ups, stretches the mind and is probably five percent of what would really happen. The governor discovers who really runs California and it's not her government.

Big Pharma's salespeople are the best, most highly trained, most seductive salespeople on earth. You won't see, for instance, a male salesperson visiting a male Physician. It will almost always be a female. She will be very good looking, extremely knowledgeable and certainly not dressed for a church service, if you get my drift. Similarly if that doctor is female, the salesman will be a hunk.

Moreover, it's not well known, but every prescription that every physician writes is recorded by the FDA. The big pharmaceutical companies have access to all of that information.

So, if a doctor is not toeing the line, that is, if he or she is not prescribing a particular medicine made by a particular pharmaceutical company, the salesman knows that and knows exactly how to present that pharmaceutical company's product.

The salesman also knows what perks to offer and to deny. If a doctor accepts any kind of perk, most of which are not illegal, the massive database knows quickly how to get to that doctor next time. Very sophisticated algorithms design sales approaches tailored precisely to individual physicians.

It's powerful.

This process of targeting physicians begins the moment a student registers for pre-med! From that day, big-pharma is watching, evaluating, learning how to sway that student upon graduation.

Perks are offered long before graduation. Free courses, subtlely slanted, are offered. Study assistance is offered. Gifts, tickets, companions, seminars to exotic places, cruises and the like are lavished upon physicians who toe the line.

It's seductive.

Doctors understand that they can make triple to quadruple their salary through kickbacks (which are never reported) just because they happen to prefer (genuinely) a particular medicine or procedure or machine.

It's no wonder that Physicians over-prescribe, prescribe inappropriate drugs and specify highly expensive procedures and scans which are not necessary.

Insurance

Oh it gets worse. There is a problem with malpractice insurance. It's very expensive. Doctors do not want to be sued for malpractice, because it could cost them their licenses and livelihoods.

For their own protection, they can and do over-prescribe medicines, procedures and tests, in the name of patient safety, but also to protect their licenses. After all, "free" medical insurance will pay for it.

We once saw a Sacramento newspaper article on page 2 that a local doctor's malpractice insurance premiums were so high that he had begun an Amway business to pay them! He did well in Amway. We knew him.

About that time, my next door neighbor, a military flight surgeon, stopped practicing medicine when he left the Air Force. He deplored socialized medicine and huge insurance requirements.

THE NUTRITION REVOLUTION

A New Form of Taxation

Insurance is not free. It is very expensive. There is no free lunch. You then I pay the policy premiums. The net result is that the whole public is taxed (by insurance companies) to pay for these unnecessary medicines, procedures and equipment. But actually most of the diseases will go away when treated holistically with proper nutrition.

That is such an important statement that I devote a new paragraph to reiterating that most of these diseases **will go away** if treated correctly with good nutrition.

One would think that the insurance companies would be all over nutritional remedies, to prevent claims. What or who restrains them?

I suspect that they increase their profits the same way that Big Pharma does. After all, if most disease disappeared, there would be little need for huge insurance premiums. Big Pharma and Big Insurance executives both might need to sell their jets and move out of their mansions.

Prevention is Better Than Healing

Don't wait for a disease to manifest itself and then cure it. That's foolish. It's also a lot harder to reverse disease than to prevent it. Diabetes, for instance, can cost you your limbs and eyes. Once they are gone, nutrition won't bring them back.

You must stay ahead of diseases such as diabetes, arthritis and cancer with proper nutrition throughout all of your life. You must prevent them and stay ahead of them.

Mothers must prevent medical problems before becoming pregnant. They must build up stores of nutrients in their bodies long before conception. The new baby needs these things within the first few days of pregnancy!

MODULE 12

Family Nutrition

If you're starting a family, what nutrition should you give your child?

If you look at infant formula, you're going to find that most of the 60 required minerals are missing. If you look at dog food, even rat food or gerbil food, you will find far more minerals than in baby food. We feed our beloved pets better than we feed our children. To be fair, very few new parents know this. They'd probably have to read this book or one by Dr. Wallach to find the truth.

Science has proven that in farm animals, all birth defects can be prevented by giving the mother proper nutrition **before** she gets pregnant.

At various stages of the pregnancy, various different trace minerals are needed to begin forming the heart, the brain, the nerves, the kidneys, liver, the palate, the fingers, etc. If those specific minerals are missing at the time that the mother's body needs them, the child has a birth defect. The drug Thalidomide probably suppressed certain minerals when it prevented limbs from forming.

It's been that way with farm animals, for half a century. Half a century ago, livestock farmers discovered they could prevent virtually all birth defects by giving the mothers proper nutrition.

This was wonderful news to them, because it prevented loss of baby animals, which was very expensive. Ever since that discovery, they feed their animals properly and they don't have problems.

I've done some computer programming for an Iowa animal feed mill. The main nutrients come in via a never-ending stream of trucks, to be stored in giant hoppers. Each mixture of food is different for different animals and birds. They make cattle food, turkey food, gerbil food, rabbit pellets, deer food, etc.

They have a few 55-gallon barrels of black powder available and according to a specific recipe, a hand scoop of that powder might go into a hopper forty feet tall and twenty feet in diameter, where mixers distribute everything evenly before the mix is pelletized. I asked what that black powder was. The manager told me it was composed of minerals.

I spoke to a rancher the other day. He confirmed that the only time he loses a calf is when a cow gets away from the herd and lives as a hermit for a long time, away from the good feed he gives his herd.

THE NUTRITION REVOLUTION

It turns out, through much-much research that the same is true of humans. Yet millions of babies are born with mineral deficiencies and birth defects. Their mothers simply were not educated to know they should store up the vitamins and minerals for a good pregnancy. They did not take the required nutrients throughout the pregnancy and did not feed them to their newborns and growing children. They thought iron and prenatal vitamins were enough.

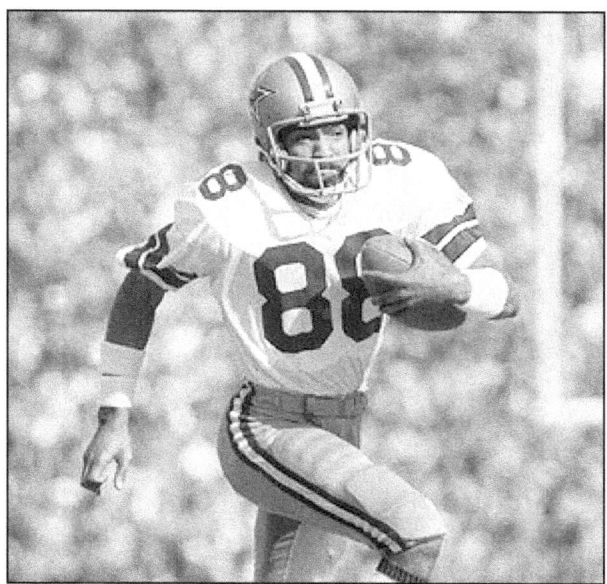

Drew Pearson, Dallas Cowboys' Wide Receiver now has become a Youngevity Brand Ambassador.

Other Diseases

As examples, several diseases were discussed above. There are other systemic, debilitating diseases to consider, in the light of nutrition.

Arthritis

Arthritis a calcium <u>deficiency</u> disease.

If your body is short of calcium, it's logical to expect the disease called osteoporosis, and its relatives. When the needs calcium, it pulls it from the bones, causing osteoporosis. As a result, the bones become porous, weak and brittle.

When the body needs calcium for such things as regulating the heart beat or helping the memory, it is going to pull it out of its boney storehouse. That means that the bone matrix remains but that calcium in the bones, which strengthens the bones, disappears. Bones become, brittle and easily fractured. That much is logical.

What is <u>illogical</u>, is that calcium deficiency causes arthritis in the joints, kidney stones, etc. What happens is the body pulls calcium from its normal stores and deposits calcium into other places such as joints and kidney stones. Then, you get arthritis, painful kidney stones and as a host of other things.

There are 147 calcium deficiency diseases, many of them not very logical but very provable and reversible.

If you have kidney stones or arthritis of its various forms, the way to get out of that trap is to add calcium to your diet!

There's more to the arthritis story, the case of calcium. Scientists, including Dr. Wallach have found that ordinary gelatin made from the bones of calves, or even chicken cartilage, especially with glucosamine sulfate or glucosamine chondroitin, will rebuild joints.

This even happens if the cartilage has been surgically removed. When a surgeon removes the cartilage in a joint, there always a few stem cells left behind, and if the body has the proper nutrient, it will rebuild the cartilage.

THE NUTRITION REVOLUTION

Taking 100% of the 90 essential nutrients and attacking the disease with glucosamine sulfate and calves gelatin, reverses and even eliminates arthritis in a few months.

Cancer is an interesting, terrible disease.

In a 2013 interview, Dr. Wallach stated that cancer is never genetic but instead it is a self-inflicted disease. Of course, nobody would intentionally give themselves cancer but the facts remain that if a woman cooks her dinner meat well done, she increases her risk of breast cancer by 462%. If she fries the dinner, it's the same.

He goes on to explain why. As noted elsewhere in this book, fats (especially vegetable oils) oxidize in a flash at frying temperatures, turning into carcinogens. So avoid fried food, period. Cook your steak rare or medium rare at low temperature. If you must use oil, make it butter only. Not even olive or coconut oil is safe. No mayonnaise, no salad dressing, no bottled oils at all.

Selenium is effective against several forms of cancer., whether or not you smoke.

As mentioned above, Dr. Wallach and Dr. Schrauser spent millions of dollars suing the FDA for the right to make that statement. The FDA lost.

THE NUTRITION REVOLUTION

I sat through a 2 ½ hour lecture by Dr. Schrauser once, while he proved that statement medically, statistically, biologically, mathematically, chemically, physically, anatomically…. He proved in 22 separate ways, that selenium is effective against cancer of the prostate, breast and lungs. With little doubt, it's effective against other forms of cancer, but he had not at the time, made those tests.

As he stated, selenium is powerful but acts much better when added to the other 90 essential nutrients.

Unfortunately for large pharmaceutical companies, selenium is a food and cannot be patented. Large pharmaceutical companies make billions upon billions of dollars from cancer every year. Cure it, and guess what! Billions and billions of dollars in profit and research grants disappear.

The ones who suffer are the poor people who get cancer, along with the rest of us who pay higher insurance premiums for unnecessary treatment, with the profits going into the medical profession.

So other than being an electrical semiconductor, what is selenium, anyhow?

It used to be considered a poison. That was because of cattle that happened to graze on ground that's extremely high in selenium. The constant exposure to the selenium caused hooves to split. The hooves were in constant contact with the mineral and absorbed massive doses.

Too much of anything is harmful – even water and oxygen. It turns out that selenium is safe, compared to many other things and it is necessary for health.

Where it doesn't exist in the land, such as areas of Western Pennsylvania, Northeastern Iowa and a specific province of China, especially where people grow most of their own food and don't import it, people have very high incidences of various diseases that go away when they get selenium.

Selenium is just a mineral. It's very common and inexpensive.

Diabetes

Diabetes is a chromium and vanadium deficiency.

It's pure coincidence but chromium and vanadium are elements added to some of the highest quality steel.

THE NUTRITION REVOLUTION

Through processes not well understood, these elements help the pancreas to regulate the amount of insulin it produces. Insulin counters blood sugar. If the sugar level is too high, then the pancreas emits additional insulin. If the level is too low, the pancreas secretes less insulin. So the pancreas has to know the current sugar level and also produce the proper amount of insulin.

The pancreas can become tired from overwork and in extreme situations, it can even fail and shut down. If that happens, or if the person was born with a defective pancreas, or if the pancreas is surgically removed, the result is instant diabetes.

Diabetes creates a high blood sugar level. That condition causes an inability of the body to heal. Sores take forever to heal, if they do at all. They can lead to gangrene and the necessity to amputate limbs. Eyesight deteriorates and blindness can result. Those are just the beginning of a long list of maladies associated with diabetes.

Fortunately, if the body gets some extra chromium and vanadium, along with the ordinary 90 essentials, diabetes reverses. The body cures itself.

Now, that's not the case with Type-I diabetes, in which the pancreas simply doesn't produce insulin. In that case, insulin injection is often a must, although some insulin pills have been made. Adding the correct amount of chromium and vanadium helps the body use injected insulin, so that less needs to be administered.

Future editions will add to this module. There is much more to relate. People who have copies of this book get free editions of this book, when they come out, for life, as long as I'm writing. I expect that to be another 50 years.

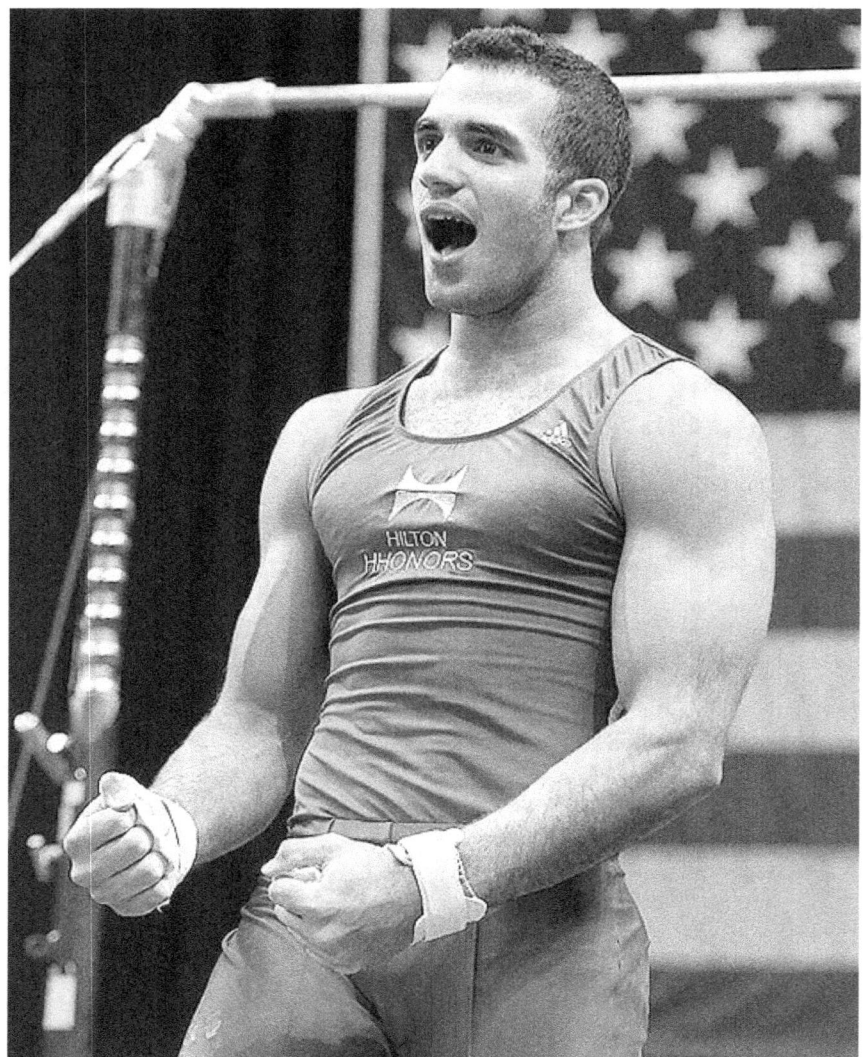

Sticking a Landing Feels Great

MODULE 13

OBTAINING THE ESSENTIAL NUTRIENTS

You Can Grow Them

Plants (and the animals that eat them) are our best source of nutrition. When that source is inadequate, supplementation is the only sensible answer.

One way to get the nutritious food we need is to grow it personally. If our back yards aren't depleted farmlands, like the tomato fields to the west of our home, the soil should be better, so one would think.

There are three major problems with that idea.

1. The earth is not homogeneous. Rocks and minerals occur in bands. Soil rich in selenium, for example, might be only ten miles from soil that has none. So even untouched back yard soil is likely to be deficient in certain minerals, and without expensive testing, one would never know which.

2. Furthermore, most back yards have been treated with various pesticides, for prettier grass. In other words, most back yard soil is poorly suited for gardening. A good gardener doesn't use it. He or she imports better soil to the food garden.

3. Many subdivisions have sprung up over depleted farmland that is worthless for crops. That's why some lawns do poorly. Even the grass has trouble finding nutrients. So owners apply fertilizers they might not put on their food plants. Most grass requires very little in the way of minerals.

Supplementing Your Soil

Bloomin' Minerals

Youngevity sells a plant supplement called Bloomin' Minerals. It's specifically for your plants. In one form, it consists of their humic shale in granule form. In liquid form, it contains the minerals derived from that shale. You just spray that on the plants about three times during the growing period.

Given the 60 minerals that you and I need, garden plants produce fruit more bountifully and with more taste than what you can get elsewhere.

Going Organic

Organic food is great (but expensive in the grocery markets.) Organic only means that the food has had no pesticides applied to it. That's all. The term Organic says nothing about the minerals in the soil. Simply don't put pesticides on your crops and they are organic.

Plants need more than just being grown 'organically.'

GMO

The term GMO stands for Genetically Modified Organisms. Here's the story.

Monsanto and some other giant companies got permission from the government to genetically modify corn, and many other crops. They unleashed a nightmare on the world.

At first, the world was concerned about GMO seeds taking over and producing plants that would crowd out native species. So Monsanto and others genetically modified the seeds so that they would grow food but would to fail to reproduce new plants. That satisfied the world's concern about rogue species but it also ensured that farmers could not grow their own seed from patented GMO strains. The farmers are bound to the seed companies.

As soon as the companies had permission to plant those seeds in test fields, gene research went further. Companies produced herbicide and pesticide resistant crops. Now, the farmer gets a boon. If he wishes, he can apply two-hundred times as much Roundup and other pesticides/herbicides to his crops. His new GMO seeds can take the punishment. Bugs and weeds cannot.

The result is higher crop yields and higher farm profits because losses to bugs and weed competition are far lower.

However, the plants grown in these conditions contain far greater levels of herbicides and pesticides than those grown before GMO seeds were produced. The result for you and me is lower food cost but there is a price. GMO foods don't digest as well as other foods. As my parents said, the "Food Value" is reduced.

Moreover, we eat those herbicides and pesticides in far greater quantities than we did before GMO came into being. Those chemicals are designed to KILL (cide) certain living things. GMO science says they do not harm people or livestock I question such statements.

Per the arsenic discussion above, everything has a therapeutic level and a toxic level. We need at least the therapeutic level and cannot tolerate the toxic level.

Some levels have not been established. Even those that have been established are for the general population, not people who are uncommonly sensitive to certain things.

THE NUTRITION REVOLUTION

Science can err. Famously, there was alleged safety of Thalidomide, a so-called safe tranquilizer given to mothers-to-be, whose children were born without limbs. More recently, we've seen science's admitted errors on salt, eggs and cholesterol.

Anything has a maximum dosage level, above which it causes bad things to happen to the body. Roundup is no different.

Consider mercury in that light. Science says that the smallest trace amount of mercury is dangerous to health, even though other science shows that our bodies absolutely must have a small, trace amount of colloidal mercury to thrive. Larger amounts, in gaseous, metallic form, are very harmful.

If scientists say that, then how could they possibly state that small amounts of Roundup and other pesticides and herbicides cause no ill effects? It's a rhetorical question. In the same breath, how could they say that up to 200 times more Roundup causes no ill effects?

Only by speaking with ignorance or a self-serving, biased, forked tongue, could they say such things. In either case, a wise person disregards such foolish statements – and grows suspicious of other statements from the same scientists.

I'm a scientist. I'm well educated. I testify that degrees and education do not substitute for the common sense God gave a goose, a bird that chooses its diet to suit its natural needs.

Small Plot Gardening

It's difficult – or at least it's financially infeasible – for a farmer to broadcast all of the essential minerals out into his vast acreage. A tiny number of specialty farmers do, but they have to charge more for their superior food.

You **can** afford to do that with a small home garden.

Here in San Diego, most people don't even own lawnmowers. We have postage-stamp lawns and concrete patios filled with chairs and a table with an umbrella. There's little extra space.

You may live in Texas or Kansas where people have yards. We have a huge lawn by San Diego standards, but it's about half the size of the Omaha lawn we left behind.

Whereas I could plant a nice garden in my San Diego yard, don't know about previous pesticides and herbicides. I chose gardens that only occupy a few square feet of space and plant them over concrete in my patio. I could even put them inside the home or garage – by providing enough light. In our temperate climate, I don't need to do that but you might consider it for a couple of reasons:

- Winter harvest and year-round harvest.
- Hiding your food supply from prying eyes, in case there's a national disaster.

A winter garden is entirely feasible. Plants that somehow know when summer and winter are, grow nicely indoors so you can fool them into producing delicious December tomatoes. You merely have a larger electric bill for the grow lights.

In San Diego, where it rarely freezes, you can probably have December beans, squash, carrots, lettuce and tomatoes outside. Just cover them when freezes threaten. Warmth from the ground or the patio will protect them.

In the mountains of Julian, California, you'll have to watch the weather more.

The key to tight spaces is to use Vertical Gardens.

Vertical Gardens

These gardens only occupy spaces from 2x2 feet to 2x4 feet to 4x4 feet. You can plant several on your patio. They are simple, quick and inexpensive to build.

My first one cost zero for materials, until I added an inexpensive dripper system. (Details below.) Okay, I did use some wood screws I already had and maybe a nickel's worth of electricity running my drill.

That doesn't count GMO-free seeds, potting soil (or dirt) and Bloomin' Minerals fertilizer. You need those anyhow.

Most of the plants are from knee to shoulder level, making harvesting easy and preventing most bugs from finding them. What a concept!

Recycle Your Water

Maintenance and watering are very easy and it's best to recycle the nutrient-rich water by pouring it back on the plants. Water lightly with the systems I'll detail below. 80% of your water will be recycled and only 20% or less will be new water. Once a week, is about right. Below, I'll detail a timed dripper system for you.

When you recycle your plants' water, you help ensure your plants have the minerals they crave. If you throw that water down the drain, you are throwing away precious minerals and soil nutrients. You wouldn't want to drink that water, because humans don't do very well on it but your plants thrive on it.

Rotating Crops

You'll discover later that if you plant your garden on a rotating basis, you can arrange for salads, beans, peas, tomatoes, carrots, radishes to appear just in time for meals year round. It's merely a matter of when you plant what, and the seed packages will tell you everything.

GMO

Seeds you plant either are GMO or they are not. Look for the label Non-GMO on the packets.

The Water Bottle Vertical Garden

Using all free materials, this garden costs nearly nothing. You might have to buy a box of screws.

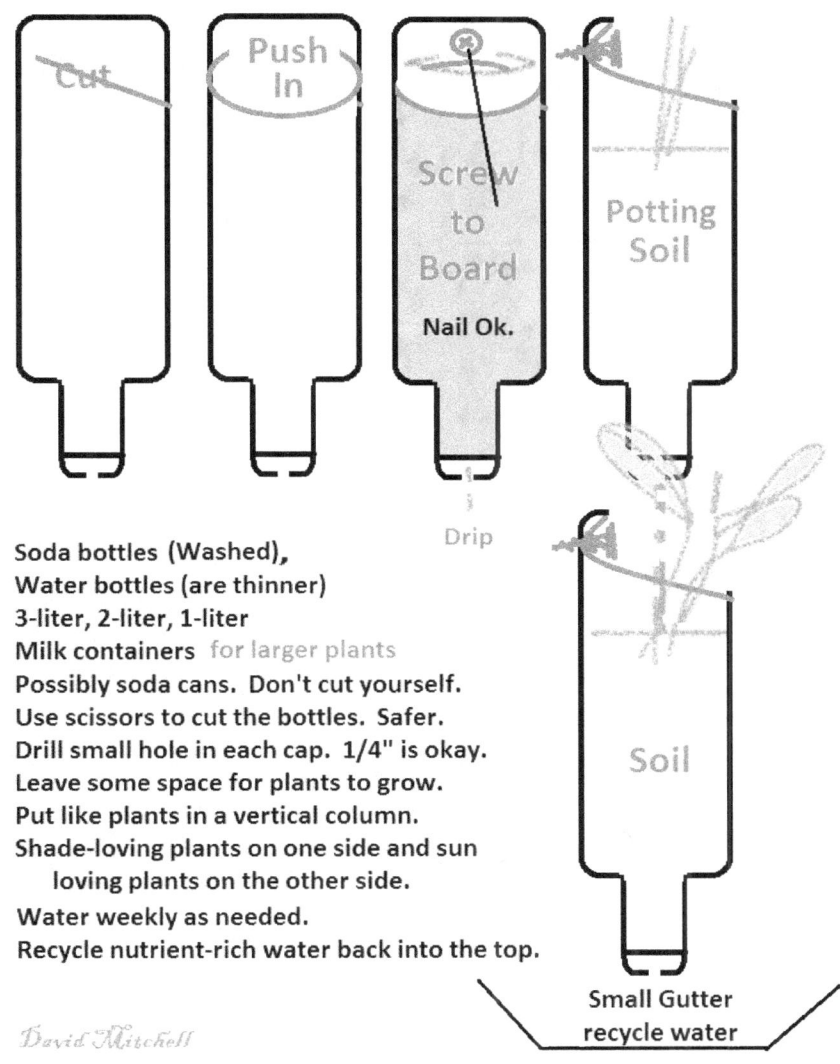

Soda bottles (Washed),
Water bottles (are thinner)
3-liter, 2-liter, 1-liter
Milk containers for larger plants
Possibly soda cans. Don't cut yourself.
Use scissors to cut the bottles. Safer.
Drill small hole in each cap. 1/4" is okay.
Leave some space for plants to grow.
Put like plants in a vertical column.
Shade-loving plants on one side and sun
    loving plants on the other side.
Water weekly as needed.
Recycle nutrient-rich water back into the top.

David Mitchell

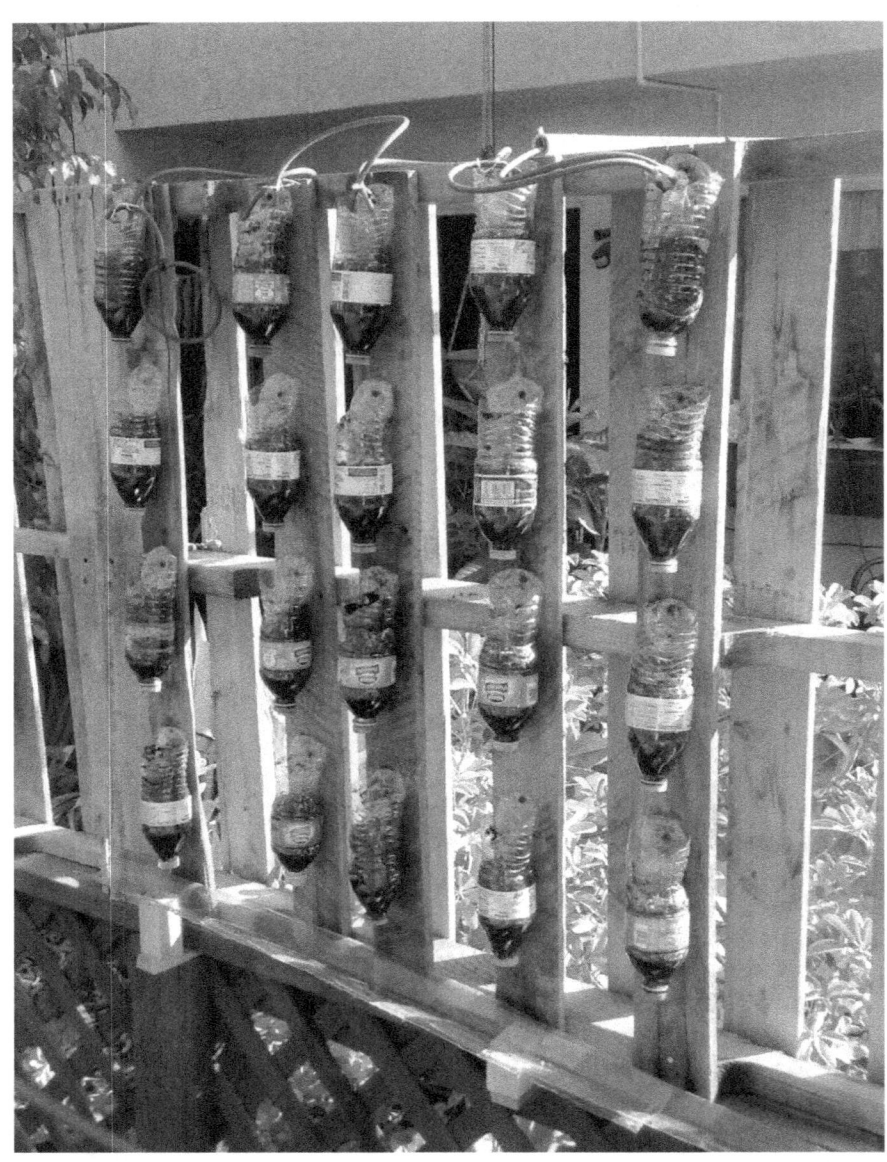

Tools

- Screwdriver or electric drill with a screwdriver bit. Give in and buy a cordless drill with a bit. It has a zillion uses. Harbor Freight has great ones for under $20. Ditto for Home Depot, Lowes, etc.

- 1/8" drill bit. It can be any size from 1/8" to 5/16".

- Scissors or shears. Don't use someone's sewing shears if you value your head.

- Possibly a claw hammer to rebuild palates.

Materials

- Scrap palates, the kind that forklifts carry.

- Scrap soda or water bottles.

- 1" wood screws, the kind with very sharp points. If you're going to rebuild palates, get some 1-1/2" long in addition.

Construction

I began with three donated, scrap palates. Stores give them away for firewood when they become too damaged to carry a lot of weight. They're perfect for a vertical garden.

I used wood from one to rebuild two palates. All I wanted was a set of vertical boards. Since a few boards were missing or broken, I salvaged boards from the third, most damaged palate.

I used recycled water bottles, with the caps. I use 2-liter and larger bottles for larger plants. Bottles last a year or two. They're free, unless you consider that you can't turn them for VAT refunds.

Plastic milk cartons are for larger plants, such as potatoes and onions.

Use a pair of scissors or kitchen shears, for the cuts. Knives work but shears are safer.

The basic idea is to cut most, not all, of the bottom out of each bottle, push the plastic inside for added strength and use a screw to attach the bottle to the palate. Make the cuts at an angle of about 20-degrees, from a point perhaps two inches up from the bottom, down to the bottom on the other side – but leave about an inch of plastic intact.

The cuts don't have to be exact. See the photos.

Invert each bottle and screw it to the palate. You can nail it but screws make it easier to replace bottles. The palate will outlast your bottles.

Below each bottle is another bottle, with bottles dripping into each other. Each one waters another so you only need to water the top row. What a concept!

The bottom bottles drip into a trough which drains into a bucket. That's the water you recycle.

Four water or soda bottles in a vertical line fill up a palate and you can have six columns, for a total of 24 bottles. Then use the other side of the palate for 24 more plants. I began with two palates, two sides each, for 96 plants and merely screwed them together in a line. I perched them on top of a low patio fence near the place where we already had a dripper system for ornamental plants.

It could hardly be simpler.

Plants need drainage. Drill each bottle cap with a small bit. You can poke a hole with a nail. I used a 1/8" drill bit but larger sizes will be fine. You are only using the cap to keep the soil in the bottle and to let the excess water drip out. You can just as easily leave caps slightly loose, or put an irregular rock in the neck of each bottle. At first, I used loose caps but found a small hole worked better.

Press potting soil into each bottle and use water to get it compacted properly. Then plant.

Add Bloomin' Minerals from Youngevity – there's nothing else like it on earth. It contains 71 minerals. Add fertilizer. Then just watch your garden grow. In two days, you will already have tiny bean and radish sprouts!

If you drink beverages in 6-paks, save the rings that hold the cans together. Don't cut the rings. Just tack them in appropriate places and let the vining plants, like beans use them for climbing. Or, ask your buddy across the street for some rings. You'll probably get an interested visitor in the process and get to know your buddy better.

The Tomato Cage Garden

Most tomatoes like to climb away from the ground, where most bugs exist. Gardeners have long used special tomato cages to enclose tomatoes planted in the ground. This is a different use for the cages.

Tools

- Pliars
- Knife
- Scissors

Materials

- Tomato Cages from a nursery or hardware store.
- Landscape Cloth. Even an old sheet would do.
- Drainage bucket.

Construction

A tomato cage is a tube of fencing wire about a foot in diameter, standing on three long wires that the gardener pokes in the ground. The fencing wire has large holes, perhaps barely small enough to keep rabbits at bay. The wire legs hold the cages erect.

Line each cage with landscaping cloth on the inside.

Give the cage a bottom to keep soil from falling through. Landscaping cloth will do.

Spread the wire legs somewhat and put the cage over a container to catch the valuable, nutrient-rich water that flows through the soil, because you will want to pour it back into the top as it collects.

Fill each cage with potting soil. You'll be using a lot more soil than with the Water Bottle garden above.

Use a sharp knife to cut an X through the landscaping cloth, everywhere you want to plant something along the sides of the cage.

You can push a seed into the hole or you can take a plant that you've already started in your window or palate garden and install it there. It's going to be very happy with the good soil and water.

Add Bloomin' Minerals and liquid fertilizer to the water.

Every few days, scoop out enough water to wet the plants and pour it into the top. Alternately, have a small pump do the watering for you, on a timer.

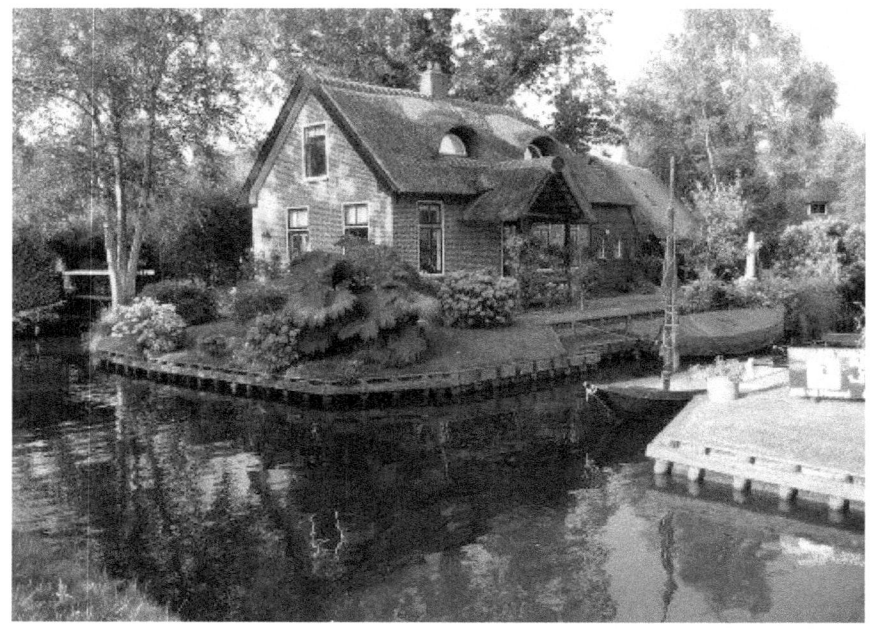

The Plastic Picnic Plate Garden

NASA engineers invented this kind of garden for the International Space Station, to save weight. It uses no soil and it grows plants faster than any other known method. I merely modified it using free and nearly-free materials.

This garden is aeroponic, not hydroponic. That means the roots grow in air, not water.

Nutrient-rich water drips over exposed roots that need no soil around them, although I start plants in soil and transfer them to the Plastic Picnic Plate Garden.

Water recycles continuously via a small pump. It is so small it can run on batteries but I plug mine in. House current is far cheaper than batteries. You can buy a solar powered pump for a lot of money. For safety, use a low voltage system, such as the ones used for sprinkler valves.

Tools

- Pliars.

- Nail, Awl, Ice Pick.

- Scissors.

Materials

- Plastic picnic plates.

- Tomato cages or wire fencing material with 2" holes or larger.

- Wire.

- Bucket.

- Pump and power supply.

- 1/4" Dripper pipe.

- Misc. Dripper fittings.

- Button Drippers, one per plate.

Construction

First, have a picnic. Okay, that's optional. Have the picnic so you can save the plastic plates. That makes them free, right? Wash them of course.

Get a tomato cage or craft the equivalent from fencing material. You can stack one tomato cage on top of another.

Some landscaping cloth forms your pots. You don't line these cages. Roll twelve inch squares of cloth into cones. Eventually, the plant roots will penetrate the cloth.

Alternately plugs of rock wool or even wads of newspaper will start your plants. When the plants are established, the newspaper will rot away but the plants will remain in place.

You can put some loose soil in each cone and plant a seed there. The soil is actually optional. Rock wool, fiberglass and similar materials work. Even cloth or newspaper would work. It wouldn't hurt to soak the material overnight in water, just in case there were some water-soluble binder chemicals in it.

THE NUTRITION REVOLUTION

Push the cones into holes in the tomato cage four or five in a circle.

Now build the watering system. Drill 7/32" holes in the centers of the plates. The holes should not be too large because the 1/4" dripper tubing should be a push fit for minimal leakage.

Build your drip system. If your plant cones are 5" above each other, cut 5" sections of 1/4" hose.

Attach button drippers and inverted plates alternately. When you're finished, the drippers will support the plates, with the drippers beneath their upside down plates. Have a feed tube at the bottom and cap the 1/4" hose at the top.

There are several ways to cap the hose. You can bend it over and secure it with a clothes pin or some wire. Alternately, you can use a T connector and attach two ends of the T with another hose so water can go nowhere.

One final button dripper goes on a very short piece of hose, just above the top plate to water that plate's plants.

Lower the drip assembly into the cage.

Just below each plate, insert a plant cone. The cones support the plate edges.

If you are planning larger plants, increase the spacing of the plates and construct a different-sized drip system.

The entire cage stands on its three legs in a 5-gallon plastic bucket, which is a few dollars at Home Depot.

The plates are there to distribute water to the roots, which are not in the center of the garden, but are around the edges. Since you want water to drip on the roots, pierce each plate's rim with a nail just above its column of plants. That way, the water always hit roots instead of falling through to the next plate. In operation, the roots will tend to find the water drips.

Keep the plates level so water goes through all of the holes more or less evenly. Use wire as necessary to level the plates.

Notice that each plate not only waters the plants directly below it, it waters other plants at the lower levels. That is perfectly okay. Lower plants get more water but that doesn't matter because this is an aeroponic system, not a soil-based system.

> *NOTE: When you over-water a plant that's in soil, the plants are susceptible to root rot, a fungus condition that destroys roots and kills plants.*

When you over-water a plant whose roots are in air, that is NOT a problem whatsoever. So your pump can supply a continuous stream of water to the plants.

A forceful jet of water can damage roots but a constant drip through a nail hole is perfect. Most pumps are designed for far more water flow than you need.

The button drippers give you the desired flow. One might be tempted to pierce the feed tube to water the plates. That could work but upper plates will starve of water. The drippers maintain constant water flow.

I have read that it's good to water during the day and not at night. Personally, I believe it's better to run the pump continuously and avoid drying the roots.

The NASA versions distribute nutrient-water through a central tube that goes up through the plates, and the disks distribute the water to the edges for the plants. The tube is pierced just above each plate. It extends down to the pump at the bottom. The piercings have to be carefully sized.

I simplified this arrangement with a standard 1/4″ tube drip system. One-gallon per hour dripper disks are above each plate, because each one supports the plate above it. The top plate has one more dripper disk immediately above it. The bottom plate is only supported by its plants and wires.

It's rather important that the plates be level for even watering, so I tie them at three points around their edges. Pull ties hold them to the cage. It's a rickety arrangement but I don't travel with it, so it works.

Investigate the dripper holes periodically to ensure they don't plug and deprive one of your plants of water.

Use liquid fertilizer that won't plug your holes. Add Liquid Bloomin' Minerals. After plants are established, spray some Bloomin' Minerals on their leaves.

THE NUTRITION REVOLUTION

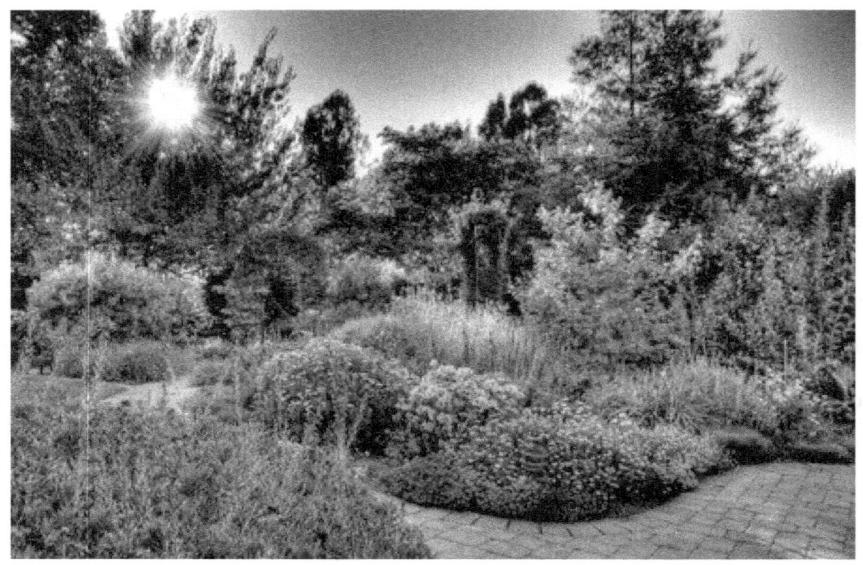

The Fencing Garden

A variant of the Tomato Cage garden uses ordinary fencing wire.

Tools

- Pliars
- Scissors
- Knife

Materials

- Bucket
- Landscape Cloth
- Fencing material
- Wire – or just clip of some fencing material for wire.

Construction

Cut 3-1/2 foot lengths* of fence and curl them into a circle, wiring the ends together.

THE NUTRITION REVOLUTION

As with the Tomato Cage garden, line with landscaping cloth, cut your X marks and plant.

> ** Pi is 3.14. the circumference of your garden is Pi x Diameter. Allow 6" more to wire things together.*
>
> *The dimensions aren't that exact. Just use 3 for Pi. So:*
>
> *If you want a 1' diameter garden, the calculation is 3 x 1 + 1/2. That comes out to 3 -1/2 foot lengths.*
>
> *It also works in inches or meters. If you want an 18" diameter garden, the length is 3 * 18 inches plus 6 inches. That comes out to be about 60" or 5'.*
>
> *If you want a garden 0.5 meters in diameter, the length is 1.5 meters plus the length of your hand.*

You use the excess 6" of wire to hook things together. Or, you can clip off some extra wire from the fence and use that.

Support the fencing wire over a drainage bucket. Periodically, transfer a quart or so of nutrient-rich water from the bucket to the top of the garden.

The Wall Garden

This garden is particularly good for starting seeds to be transplanted elsewhere, but you can leave the plants right there. It is a bit more complicated than the other gardens but it is also more versatile.

Tools

Electric drill.

1/4" drill bit.

Bit to drive the screws.

Hammer.

Wire cutters.

Pliars. They often have wire cutting ability.

Materials

Two 4' lengths of 2x4 lumber. 2x2 will do. This is for the frame's horizontal width. You can also make it wider or narrower. Do not use "treated" lumber because the green lumber contains arsenic and the blue is suspicious. Cypress lumber will not rot. Cedar lasts a long time. Pine lasts several years and may be the cheapest in the long run.

Two 5' lengths of 2x4 lumber. 2x2 is okay. This is for the frame's vertical pieces. You can make it taller or shorter.

Tacking strips measure about 1/8" by 1". They are optional to hold the cloth and wire in place. They will tack to the frame pieces all around.

The fence wire does a good job of holding the cloth. Tacking strips, secured with screws, make it easier to rebuild the assembly in future years.

Lengths of landscape cloth to fit the frame all around, on both sides, wrapping. A 4' x 5' garden would require 8-1/2 feet of 5' cloth.

Lengths of wire fence to wrap around the cloth. The length is the same as the cloth. The holes should be at least 2″ wide and at least 2″ tall. Fencing should be rust resistant. Galvanized* is okay. Plastic coated is even better.

> *Galvanizing is a process of dipping in zinc to prevent the underlying iron from rusting. Chemically, the zinc goes first as a sacrificial material. When it's gone the iron starts to rust. Our bodies love zinc, with the exception of the rare few who are sensitive to it.*

Rock wool to fill a space 3″ x 4′ x 5′ for the 4′ x 5′ garden. That would be 5 cubic feet. The rock wool will be compressed somewhat. Rock wool is used as wall insulation.

Larger or smaller frames would mean less or more rock wool.

16 deck screws 3-1/2 or 4″ Long. They should be rust resistant. There are many kinds of rust resistant screws. You can probably get a small box of screws cheaper than buying 16 individual ones.

Box of 1″ deck screws, also rust resistant. You can use nails but screws let you change the cloth and interior rock wool more easily in a year or two.

Construction

Build a frame or 2x2 or 2x4 lumber to stand by itself or to lean against something else. Almost any size frame will do. Mine measures 4' wide by 5' tall and I found 2x4 lumber cheaper than 2x2.

For better strength, cut the 2x4 ends at 45-degree angles and screw them together with four screws per joint. Offset the screws slightly so one doesn't hit another and split the wood.

Don't be tempted to use "green wood" which resists rot but which contains poisonous salts. You don't want your plants contaminated.

! !

Ask your lumber person for safe wood. There is a "blue wood" but I don't know what chemical they use to prevent it from rotting. It's supposed to be safe. Untreated wood is obviously safer.

I prefer the new plastic decking material, which is more expensive but which does not rot.

Cedar and redwood are long-lasting. Cypress will never rot. Pine will last several years and overall may be the cheapest.

Nobody cares about knots or imperfections, so construction grade material is fine. You can paint it for added protection but of course don't use lead based paint, even if you can find the poisonous stuff.

Tack landscape cloth on one side of the frame but not around to the other side yet. Drive a few screws or staples if that makes the job easier.

Tack the fencing over the landscape cloth, again on one side only. I use tacking strips and screws for easier disassembly later.

Turn it over and overfill it with rock wool. Push the wool in to compact it.

Wrap the landscape cloth around the other side.

Wrap and tack the fencing to the other side.

I use plastic coated wire, because I have some.

Cut an X-shaped hole where you want to put a plant. Push a seed in there (not too far) or make a plug for the seed or plant a pre-established plant.

For water distribution, drill many holes in the top and bottom. I drill ¼" holes every two inches.

THE NUTRITION REVOLUTION

You can see that the top and bottom boards are going to be wet most of the time. For this reason, I prefer aluminum or one of the new plastic decking materials for the frame, especially the top and bottom. Wood that is well-coated with Urethane or Epoxy is a good alternative. Go so far as to coat the interiors of your drip holes. A syringe filled with Urethane or Epoxy, or some pipe cleaners will do the job.

You need a trough at the bottom that can collect water into a bucket. I make troughs out of corrugated fiberglass roofing material, that wavy stuff. I cut it with a Dremel tool. It splits if you try to shear it.

Recycle that water into the top because it is highly nutritious to plants.

You need a trough at the top which you can put water. For this, you can merely attach a strip of wood on each side of the top, extending up a half inch or so. I used tacking strips for the upper trough walls.

Planting

Plants need these things:

- Water
- Light
- Nutrition
- Air

Water

Water weekly. First, add a small amount of fertilizer to the nutrient-rich water that has drained through your plants and follow up with fresh water.

It's easy to tell if you are over-watering or under-watering. Just look at your runoff bucket. If the amount of water there is increasing, you are over-watering. If the bucket is running dry, you are under-watering. Excess water automatically drains through the plants and falls out the bottom.

THE NUTRITION REVOLUTION

My preference is to water after a family dinner on the patio. After I've drained my water glass, I scoop a glassful of runoff water from the bucket, heavy in fertilizers and minerals, and dump as much as I can into the top plants of each row. They will drain down into the lower plants and I don't have to water those. I do anyhow, because I know I can't over-water. The drain holes in the caps ensure each plant gets the right amount of water.

I do that about once a week and it might take ten minutes. I get to look at the new greenery that way. If anything has not sprouted, I drop a new seed in that bottle.

I have a dripper system and rarely use it because water from it has no nutrients. That water tends to leach minerals out of the soil, to be captured by the bucket. When my bucket runs low, I turn the drippers on and fertilize at that time so the plants always have plenty of fertilizer and minerals. Then when my bucket is getting full after a week, I turn it off and return to manual watering.

Some people prefer rain water because it is devoid of chlorine and fluorine, which some plants won't tolerate well. I disagree.

I don't recommend rain water because it probably fell on the asphalt roof and drained off. I have no idea what chemicals the shingle makers put in their asphalt or fiberglass shingles, but their roof making doesn't have to be fit for human consumption, so I don't use rain water. If I had a tile or cement tile roof, that might be a different matter. There's yet another issue.

Storing rain water is problematic. Even if loosely covered, it becomes a breeding ground for mosquitoes. The West Nile Virus is spread by mosquitoes and you certainly don't want to catch that one. It's such a debilitating disease that our county has a well-funded initiative to eliminate standing water and mosquitoes.

We tried pouring cooking oil on the water in our barrels. That didn't work. It got smelly and mosquitoes got in anyhow.

Jason Richardson solved the mosquito problem. Use ordinary window screens. The rain water goes through the screen easily but the mosquitos can't get in to lay eggs. That presents another problem – how to remove the water.

THE NUTRITION REVOLUTION

Robert Mach solved that one. He works at Home Depot. They sell a small pump whose shank fits into a cordless drill. It's their least expensive pump. It uses garden hose, so buy a hose and cut it in two. The female end of the hose goes on the pump. Unfortunately, the manufacturer put two male ends on the pump so you need to buy an adapter if you're going to use the other end of the hose. An adapter might cost less than a second hose.

Make a hole in the screen for the hose and seal it well with duct tape to keep out wily mosquitoes. They smell your water and will try to get in to lay eggs.

A framed window screen can lay on top of your rain barrel. Alternately, you can use some calking or silicone rubber to glue screening material to the rim.

When you need water, pump it into a bucket and carry it to your plants.

We considered another way to get water out. You can buy a spigot at Home Depot that you can install at the bottom of the barrel. If the barrel is on a stand, you can drain water from the barrel into your tote bucket. If not, you can pump it into your bucket via the hose and the spigot. We rejected the idea because it costs more.

If you have a water softener, it probably removes most of the chlorine and fluorine.

It doesn't make sense to buy a water softener just for your garden. You might buy bottled water for your garden but I don't.

Tap water is perfectly okay. It's already pure enough for human consumption and the garden plants purify it further before putting it into their cells. They are extremely good at purifying contaminated water. For example, coconut water is sterile enough to substitute for blood plasma in wartime. Jungle vines and exposed roots of some trees produce pure water for the thirsty. Tap water is far cleaner than what plants are accustomed to getting from the ground. Moreover, tap water has calcium and other minerals the plants love.

When watering plants in the ground, too little water dries them out and too much leads to root rot, one of several fungi that destroy roots and thus the plants. These, on the other hand, are hydroponic and aeroponic gardens. Root rot is rarely a problem, except that when you use potting soil, the fungi can be in the potting soil. For that reason, gardeners ensure good soil drainage.

Use a dripper system and adjust its little valves so each plant gets the right amount of water. You can water manually and should recycle your runoff water that way. Also ensure excellent drainage so the roots stay moist but not wet when in soil.

THE NUTRITION REVOLUTION

Light

Typical gardens get about six hours of effective sunlight a day. The sun is up far longer, of course, but plants shade each other. Early morning and evening hours are usually full of shade.

Find the sunniest place in your yard and install your garden there so one side gets morning sun and the other gets afternoon sun. A wall garden would be aligned North-South. Or, have sun-loving plants on the south side and shade loving plants on the north side of an East-West garden.

A pocket compass can tell help you find North, or you can look for the North Star (Polaris) at night. Find the Big Dipper. Its outer cup stars point to Polaris and on the other side of the North Star is Cassiopeia, the big W in the sky. If you know your latitude in degrees, the North Star is that many degrees above the horizon. If that's too much trouble, use a road map and estimate your personal North from that. Or just notice where the sun is at noon. That's due South.

Nutrition

There are two nutrients you will probably want to add to your water. One is Bloomin' Minerals from Youngevity and the other is a good liquid fertilizer.

Don't over-fertilize. The packages tell you how much to use.

Air

Plants use carbon dioxide from the air and through photosynthesis release oxygen. Ordinary air is fine for them.

Temperature

Don't let plants freeze because ice crystals burst their cells and kill them. Some plants have built-in anti-freeze but most die when the weather freezes.

Similarly, don't burn the plants with too much heat. Even well-watered plants wither when it gets too hot. If it's relatively comfortable for you, the plants will be okay.

If the weather will be too cold, cover your plants with something to keep out the wind. Sheets may do the trick. Foam cones will save ordinary tomato plants from frost several degrees below freezing. They work because the ground is not frozen. It is perhaps 10-30 degrees warmer than the chilling air. If you cover plants, the ground keeps them warm.

If the weather will be too hot, simply shade the plants from direct sun by whatever means if feasible.

When I was growing up, I heard on the radio that it was 100 degrees in the shade. I asked my dad what that would be in terms of degrees in the sun. I was always asking questions like that. He gave me a thermometer. Shortly afterward, I came back in, sweating, saying the thermometer had maxed out at 120 and it was hotter than that. My tomatoes out back didn't mind the heat at all. I won second place with them at the county fair that year.

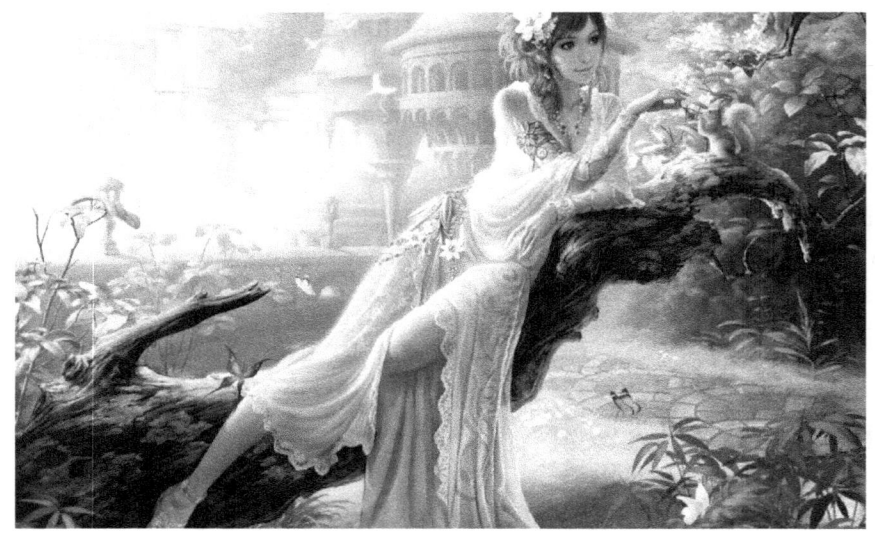

Your Planting Schedule

You can live beautifully with nature and have year-round harvests. Merely plant at the right times.

Seed packets tell you how long it will be before you can harvest any given plant. So if you want peas during July, for instance, plant your peas that many days early.

Then if you want more peas during August, plant more peas four weeks later. Or you can plant half as many peas every two weeks. Do keep track of what you plant where.

It's the same for all plants. Look up the time from planting to harvest for each crop and plant early. It's just like planning a meal. You wouldn't pour the milk and then put the roast in the oven. Plan backwards from the desired outcome.

A planting schedule ensures a nice selection of vegetables all year round but it does require constant planting. You can plant for excess, to sell or trade at the farmer's market.

In an economic crisis, food will become extremely valuable.

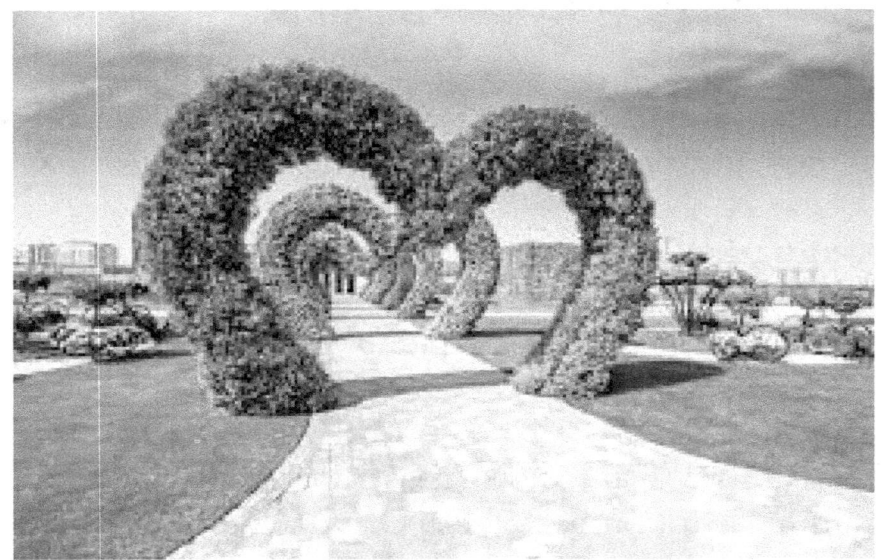

Tips to Live and Love Well Past 100

1. Avoid GMO foods. Pay extra money for good food.

2. Choose Organic foods. Pay extra money for good food.

3. If you garden, fertilize fully, using Bloomin' Minerals.

4. Supplement your diet with the 90 Essential Nutrients in liquid and capsule form. Pay extra money and consume what your body needs.

If you do those things, you will:

5. Live longer.

6. Live younger.

7. Have superior energy.

8. Enjoy greater stamina.

9. Get more done.

10. Enjoy life more.

11.Prosper more.

In general, you will Live More. And Better. And Younger.

You're worth the price.

Summary

1. Humans need 60 minerals, 16 vitamins, 12 amino acids and at least 2 fatty acids, total of 90, to thrive.

2. Our soils are depleted so farmlands can no longer produce the high quality food we need.

3. Even pristine, undepleted soils are deficient in various minerals because the earth's crust is not homogenous. Minerals occur in bands of rocks. As evidence, miners seek concentrations of minerals to make mining more profitable. This means that farmlands devoid of particular minerals may be only a hundred feet or a hundred miles from soils containing plenty of those minerals.

4. Bottom land, that is land composed of silt from mountains, and plains brought in by rivers, is the best farmland.

5. If farmers could supplement their acreage, profitably, they would. However, such full supplementation is prohibitively expensive.

6. Plants need minerals to make vitamins and amino acids. Fish need minerals to make essential fatty acids.

7. People must supplement their diets with the 90 essential nutrients because they cannot buy adequately nutritious foods at any reasonable cost.

8. It's feasible for individual families to grow much of their produce in high quality environments, year round. They supplement their potting soil with the 60 essential minerals and their plants do the rest.

9. One can grow more produce in vertical gardens than horizontal, while keeping most bugs at bay.

10. Families can earn good livings by spreading the word about nutrition. We do and we know thousands of others who do just that.

Nutrition News

I invite you to <u>Nutrition News</u>, our periodical designed to help you live longer. It's cost-free but it's not public. I must have your permission to send it to you.

To do that, all you have to do is one of the following:

1. Send me an email with your name and email address. I'll see to it that you're enrolled. My address is David@DM1.US. Or,

2. Do the same, except Email to NutritionNews@DM1.US. Or,

3. Write a letter to me at 13017 Trail Dust Ave., San Diego, CA 92129. Or,

4. Visit DM1.US and find the Nutrition News form. Just list your confidential email address and name there and Join the Family. Or,

5. Visit MKTG.ORG and find the Nutrition News form there and Join the Family. Or,

6. Call me at 858-538-2911 and I'll set it up. Or,

7. Find my Nutrition News BLOG at WordPress. Or,

8. Find me on Twitter, Facebook, Linked In, etc. and seek a link to the Join Nutrition News form.

I've tried to make it easy. It really is easy to find me and it really is easy to

LIVE LONG IN PROSPERITY AND GREAT HEALTH.

MODULE 14

YOUNGEVITY PRODUCTS

We want everyone healthy. No exceptions.

Wholesale Only.

To that end, we make all Youngevity products available at straight wholesale prices. You can pay more but you can't legally pay less. Everything comes brand-new, direct from Youngevity's warehouse to you at the same prices we pay for our personal products.

Phone-In Orders

When you phone us, usually, we pay or arrange for no sales tax and sometimes we can pay shipping. That's only for phone-in orders. We want to talk to you and get to know you as friends, not merely people who order products. We talk to Youngevity for you and arrange for them to ship to you directly.

Online Orders

We recognize that some people prefer to order online and that's perfectly okay with us too. We offer products on our website DM1.US, also at strict wholesale prices. You pay shipping and sometimes pay sales tax.

Payment

We use PayPal, which also accepts credit cards.

We will gladly accept your personal check or money order. If you're local, we even accept cash and give you an invoice of course. We merely put your money in our bank account and order your products on our credit card. Youngevity doesn't accept personal checks but as a courtesy, we do.

Our address is:

13017 Trail Dust Ave., San Diego, CA 92129

Direct from Youngevity Orders

If you prefer to order directly from Youngevity, that's okay too. They only sell to Associates ($10 one time to become one) and Preferred Customers (No Charge to be one.) You get an ID number and they will take your card and ship it directly at Wholesale. They always charge shipping and sales tax. Shipping is $6.50 minimum or 8% of the wholesale value of the contents. Tax depends on your locality. It's 8% to 10% for most places.

Literature

Youngevity doesn't sell books or CDs, due to conflict of interest and FDA rules. Wellness Publications handles all of Dr. Wallach's publications, as well as publications by other eminent people. You can reach Wellness through us or directly at 800-755-4656. They will take normal forms of payment. Their website is

http://DrJWallach.Com.

This book, "Nutrition Revolution" is available In Full Color for $39.97 at:

http://Amazon.Com,

http://MachBooks.Com,

http://WillDMitchell.Com and

http://DM1.US.

It's a bit pricey because it's printed on color paper. It is also available in Kindle format for less.

Product Selection Simplified

With a score of Healthy Body Packs, Youngevity has something for nearly everyone, covering some 900 diseases. Navigation can be difficult so here are some simplifications worked out by Dr. Wallach and our friend Todd Smith.

THE NUTRITION REVOLUTION

One basic Healthy Body Start Pack is what a 100# person needs every month, to stay healthy. For instance, I weigh 191# so I consume two a month (unless I get forgetful about it.)

The Healthy Body Start Pack comes in two flavors because one of its components, Beyond Tangy Tangerine comes in two flavors: Original Tangerine and Citrus Peach Fusion 2.0.

The two are basically equivalent. It's a matter of taste, but the 2.0 costs $3 more than the Original and uses a greater variety of fruits and vegetables in its manufacture. We like original's taste better but about half of our friends like the 2.0 Peach flavor better.

The Healthy Body Start Pack is the basis for most of the other Healthy Packs. For instance, if you have blood sugar problems, Dr. Wallach adds Sweet-Eze to the Healthy Body Start Pack. That creates the Healthy Body Blood Sugar Pack – in the two versions mentioned above: tangerine and peach.

The process is similar for Weight Loss, Bones and Joint problems, as well as Heart and Brain problems. The Packs are named:

- Healthy Body Start Pack.
    - o For people already in good health.
    - o This pack contains Beyond Tangy Tangerine (Original) or BTT 2.0 Citrus Peach Fusion, functionally the same product in two flavors.
    - o The pack also contains Osteo-Fx, the only liquid calcium source that is 97% bio-available.

- o Rounding out the package, it contains Essential Fatty Acids, importantly Omega 3 and Omega 6.

- Healthy Body Blood Sugar Pack.

  - o For people with high or low blood sugar. This pack helps the pancreas adjust blood sugar to optimal levels.

  - o This pack adds Sweet-Eze to the Healthy Start Pack.

- Healthy Body Bone and Joint Pack

  - o For people with various hard tissue problems. Hard Tissues include the bones, cartilage and the collagen that holds softer tissues together.

- Healthy Body Brain and Heart Pack

  - o For people with various soft tissue conditions. Soft tissues include the brain and heart, of course, but also the various organs and muscles in the body.

  - o This pack adds Gluco-Gel and CM Crème. The Gluco-Gel supports joint health and even helps regrow cartilage in the joints. CM Crème is a safe analgesic crème to rub on anything that hurts, including sore joints and even sore muscles.

- Healthy Body Weight Loss Pack

  - o For people desiring to lose weight down to their optimum.

     o This pack adds A.S.A.P. for powerful weight loss. These are drops absorbed under the tongue. They cause the body to burn adipose (brown) fat as fuel. This is the kind of fat that is hardest to lose and is the most dangerous.

Some people want all powders, for easier traveling.

Others want to ensure there are no products derived from shellfish or tuna.

Others want everything in liquid form, or at least in powders that can be mixed with water or juice – that is, no pills or capsules.

Others want absolutely no sweeteners in their products.

There are packs for all of those contingencies.

Specialty Packs

You may hear about the Pig Pack or the Pig Arthritis Formula, Those legacy items are available for people who love them but the Healthy Body Bone and Joint Pack is equivalent. The Ferret Fat Pack is replaced by the Healthy Body Weight Loss Pack. We can supply the ingredients of the Stud Horse Pack. It's the Healthy Body Start Pack plus Prost-fx for reproductive health.

All components of the packs are available separately. Buying a pack usually saves a few dollars.

If you need a unique specialty pack, you can get the deed done.

For example, if you have bone and joint problems and also have blood sugar problems, you shouldn't go to the expense of two packs: (1) bone and joint and (2) blood sugar. Doing that would double up on three products: Osteo-Fx, Tangerine and EFA. Your best choice would be to amedd Gluco-Gel and CM Crème to the Healthy Body Blood Sugar Pack.

Similarly, if you have kidney failure and diabetes, Dr. Ma Lan recommends the Healthy Body Blood Sugar Pack plus Ultimate Daily.

Call me. Dr. Wallach and Dr. Ma Lan trust me to help you correctly. 858-538-2911. 9-9 Pacific time.

When to be Cautious

It would be economically prohibitive to overdose on these particular minerals and vitamins. They are exceedingly safe. There are rare situations in which one should take care, however.

For example, if you are under a physician's care for a replacement kidney or other organ, you must continually watch your immune system for signs that the body is rejecting the organ. Dr. Wallach's products strengthen your immune system, so if you have a donor kidney or other organ, it's possible that the immune system will become too strong. You don't want to risk organ rejection, so consult with your physician.

THE NUTRITION REVOLUTION

The minerals, vitamins, amino acids and fatty acids are still required in your diet for long life. You would want to be careful about your total immunity, because of the possibility of organ rejection. You definitely don't want to lose that new organ.

Our panel of physicians also can help you. I can put you in touch with the right ones. They are Very good.

Catalogue

A book like this cannot possibly keep up with everything in the Youngevity catalogue but below are the most important items, taken directly from the Youngevity catalogue.

To browse the complete set of products, somewhere between 500 and 1,000 of them, go to http://DM1.US.

Click the button to Shop Youngevity.

In the next page of that website, click the central All Products button or select a category like Healthy Packs from those in the oval. You can browse all of the ingredients, check wholesale and retail prices, etc. Disregard the retail prices; they're only there for reference. DM1.US always sells at Wholesale.

I can't guarantee the prices of course, because Youngevity does have to make price changes on occasion, as ingredient costs rise and fall. Yes, if ingredient costs fall, Youngevity reduces prices!

As prices change, I'll revise this book and be happy to email you a new copy, free. I need your up-to-date email, of course. You can send it to me here: David@DM1.US

http://DM1.US lists the current prices.

Youngevity Customer Service is 800-982-3197 8-5 Pacific, weekdays and you can call me at 858-538-2911 or 858-538-9455 from 9-9 Pacific time, except Sunday AM when I put my cell phone on vibrate.

Payment

You can pay via PayPal if you have a PayPal account or even if you don't, you can enter your credit card into the PayPal site. It is VERY secure and nobody but PayPal will ever see your card. My daughter used to work for PayPal Security and we're very impressed with them.

Shipment

Youngevity will ship directly to you from their headquarters / warehouse / factory at 2400 Boswell Road, Chula Vista, CA, just south of San Diego, California.

They use UPS or US Post Office, your choice. If you are accepting delivery to a P.O. box, it's better to specify Post Office because otherwise, UPS hands the package off to the Post Office, incurring a couple days of added shipping time.

Shipping takes 1-5 days but that doesn't count Sundays, so make it six days. Add a day or two for Youngevity to fill the order and you get about a week. Eight days is not uncommon. Winter storms or the rare truck breakdown can add a day or two.

Expedited shipping, even overnight, is available but expensive. They will ship anywhere in the country, even to your Aunt Essie many states removed from where you live. If you're going on vacation in Yosemite, for example, they will ship to where you will be staying. Just say where you want it delivered and be sure you'll be there to take delivery.

International shipping is available through several means. There probably are taxes and customs charges to pay at the receiving end.

Guarantee

Youngevity guarantees everything for 30 days, no questions asked. If a product is bad or damaged, they extend the guarantee much longer for you. Sometimes, they charge an 8% restocking fee for returns but never if there was any problem with the order.

> *Once when they sent the wrong products to someone we know, they merely told her to keep or return the item at her option, on their dime, and they express shipped the correct items the same day. She got a free $42 canister of the wrong product. It was just a packing error.*

About twice a year for our customers, a package gets lost because UPS mis-delivers it. In that case, Youngevity <u>immediately</u> forwards the replacement and several months later receives reimbursement or the product back from UPS. If a lost product arrives after you've received the replacement, the easiest thing for you to do is refuse the second shipment. If you incur a shipping expense due to a Youngevity or shipper error, Youngevity will refund that money.

Automatic Shipping

They can arrange monthly Auto-Shipping if you want, and in that case, shipping is free for orders totalling $50 or more. They charge your card just before shipping the product.

Customer Service

Their customer service people are kind, bilingual, diligent and knowledgeable. You can call them from 7am to 5pm, Pacific Time, Weekdays. Their number is 800-982-3189 or 800-982-3197. If ever you have difficulty, my number is 858-538-2911 and we can arrange a 3-way call. If you have extremely tough questions, they can put you in touch with various managers and doctors who have the answers. So can I.

Prices

We're all subject to inflation and occasionally (hooray) deflation. I do my best to keep up with prices.

You can go to DM1.US, click the Shop Youngevity button and on the next page click the central button to go to All Youngevity products. What you find there is accurate.

SELECTED SCIENTIFIC STUDIES

Cancer and Tangy Tangerine (From Clemson University)

CANCER CELLS

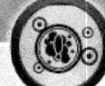

Cancer is categorized as a class of over 100 diseases. The diseases and conditions are so varied because the pathology of cancer begins with a single abnormal cell. The body is made up of trillions of living cells that grow, divide, and die in an orderly fashion. Deep within the cell, in its DNA, this process is tightly regulated. However, when cells become cancerous, the cells do not divide or behave in a healthy or orderly manner. Instead, unhealthy cells, the cells that are supposed to follow a natural programmed cell death, begin to multiply uncontrollably. These damaged cells with their improper functioning DNA, begin to breakdown and release components that can promote the spread of disease. The cell is the basic, fundamental unit of the body, its organs and systems. When the body becomes filled with cells that are not functioning properly, one can understand how this could be devastating and catastrophic to the body.

HUMAN CANCER CELL LINE RESULTS

Human Cells Lines: Cancer is categorized by the area in which the abnormal growth and cells that contain damaged DNA are present. The true cause of cancer has not been found, and, through research, it seems to be a very complex and multi-perspective position. Therefore, evaluation of how to safely eradicate cancer cells has been the immediate focus; due to the current therapies that are not discriminatory and eliminate both healthy and unhealthy cells. Cell lines can be cultivated from any areas of the body susceptible to cancer. The following studies have taken cell lines from the colon, liver, stomach, and breast; each of these cells lines was cancerous. A normal colon cell line was also taken to be a control sample.

STUDY ONE (CYTOTOXICITY ACTIVITY AGAINST CELL LINES):

Beyond Tangy Tangerine® and Ultimate Classic® were administered to the various cell lines, normal and cancerous, to assess the survival rates of the cells. First, both products were given to healthy colon cells to assess whether there was a significant amount of death of healthy cells. Next, both products were given to each unhealthy or cancerous cell lines of the colon, liver, stomach, and breast to assess whether there was a significant amount of death of each individual type of cancer cell.

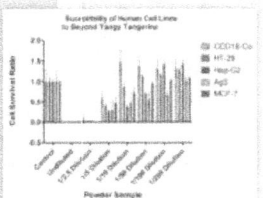

Results: When Beyond Tangy Tangerine® and Ultimate Classic® were administered to healthy human colon cells, there was no significant death of healthy human cells compared to cancerous colon cells. When exposed to Ultimate Classic®, there was a 95% reduction in cancerous colon cells, 65% of cancerous liver and stomach cells, and 30% of cancerous breast cells. When exposed to Beyond Tangy Tangerine®, there was a 60% reduction of cancerous colon cells, 65% of cancerous liver and stomach cells, and 30% of cancerous breast cells. Both products were administered at levels above and below the recommended levels, the percentages above directly relate to the recommended dosage of both products.

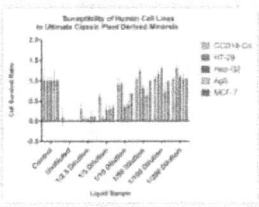

STUDY TWO (MTS CELL PROLIFERATION ASSAY):

All the cancerous cell cultures were washed with saline and given fresh media or growing environment after being subjected to both products; Beyond Tangy Tangerine® and Ultimate Classic®. Each cell line was evaluated at 24 hours post-treatment to see if there was any proliferation of cancerous cells. Survival rates of treated cells were compared to that of the untreated cells.

Result: Beyond Tangy Tangerine® and Ultimate Classic® both exhibited efficient inhibition on proliferation of cancerous cells at the recommended dosage levels. The assays, or evaluations, were carried out multiple times, sextuplicates (n=6), to confirm the results. Both products showed there was inhibition of the growth of more cancerous cells, preventing further malignant multiplication and growth of unhealthy cells.

AL International (JCOF) Announces Results of Youngevity Clinical Research Studies Performed by Clemson University – Institute of Nutraceutical Research

San Diego, CA – January 25, 2013 – Youngevity Essential Life Sciences (www.youngevity.com), a wholly-owned subsidiary of AL International, Inc. (OTC Pink: JCOF) (www.alintjcof.com), a fast growing, innovative, global direct marketer of healthy lifestyle and nutritional products and gourmet fortified coffee, announced today the exciting results of a series of clinical research studies performed by Clemson University – Institute of Nutraceutical Research ("INR").

The INR is a national leader in nutritional research and one of the most highly regarded organizations in the field of phytonutrients, vitamins and minerals. The goals of the INR are to develop greater confidence in product quality, effectiveness, and enhance consumer demand for quality nutraceutical products.

The clinical studies were performed to identify the potential benefits of Youngevity's signature core products, Beyond Tangy Tangerine and Ultimate Classic. Youngevity's mission was to truly understand and clinically substantiate the health promoting benefits of these two products. Individually, each product targets specific areas, needs, and nutritional deficiencies of the body.

Multiple studies were recommended by Clemson University scientists to provide a comprehensive evaluation of the Youngevity products. Specific biomarkers were chosen to study in the areas of safety, inflammation, and when Beyond Tangy Tangerine and Ultimate Classic were administered to cancer cell cultures.

Youngevity Clinical Research Study Highlights:

- Dietary supplement safety is the most highly regarded aspect of any of the Youngevity various products and has become synonymous with the Youngevity name and brand. Although Youngevity only uses nutrients that are absolutely needed by the body and in forms that are highly bioavailable, Youngevity felt it was important to show empirically the range and degree of safety through looking at (3) factors – Genotoxicity, Anti-Genotoxicity, and Anti-Mutagenicity. The results of the experiments showed that Beyond Tangy Tangerine and Ultimate Classic at various concentrations did not show any genotoxicity.

- When Beyond Tangy Tangerine and Ultimate Classic were administered to healthy human cell lines; they did not induce or create any inflammatory response in levels above and below the recommended dosage. Beyond Tangy Tangerine and Ultimate Classic showed inflammation protective properties and heightened the body's protective responses to possible inflammation.

- When Beyond Tangy Tangerine and Ultimate Classic were administered to healthy human colon cells; there was no significant death of healthy human cells compared to cancerous colon cells. Ultimate Classic killed 95% of cancerous colon cells, 65% of cancerous liver cells, 65% of cancerous stomach cells, and 30% of cancerous breast cells. Beyond Tangy Tangerine killed 60% of cancerous colon cells, 65% of cancerous liver and stomach cells, and 30% of cancerous breast cells.

- Beyond Tangy Tangerine and Ultimate Classic both exhibited efficient inhibition on proliferation of cancerous cells at the recommended dosage levels. Both products showed there was inhibition of the growth of more cancerous cells, preventing further malignant multiplication and growth of unhealthy cells.

The Clemson University studies have provided Youngevity greater confidence in their products, scientist, formulators, and manufacturing processes and helped to understand some of the pathways the Youngevity products may be working through in order to provide these benefits.

THE NUTRITION REVOLUTION

AL International CEO, Steve Wallach, adds, "At Youngevity we have always sought to provide high quality and safe products, these studies have added to the assurance we have in all of the Youngevity products."

About Youngevity(R) Essential Life Sciences

Youngevity Essential Life Sciences (www.youngevity.com), headquartered in San Diego, CA, is a nutrition and lifestyle-related services company dedicated to promoting vibrant health and flourishing economics. Founded in 1997 by Drs. Joel Wallach, DVM, ND, and Ma Lan, MD, as AL Global, Inc., the company adopted the name Youngevity in 2006. Youngevity is the only direct selling company to have a qualified FDA Health Claim. Dr. Wallach's work has been published in more than 70 peer-reviewed and referenced scientific journals and books.

About AL International

AL International, Inc. (OTC Pink: JCOF) (www.alintjcof.com) is a fast-growing, innovative, multi-dimensional company that offers a wide range of consumer products and services, primarily through person-to-person selling relationships that comprise a "network of networks." The company also is a vertically-integrated producer of the finest coffees for the commercial, retail and direct sales channels. AL International was formed after the merger of Youngevity Essential Life Sciences (www.youngevity.com) and Javalution Coffee Company in the summer of 2011.

Safe Harbor Statement

This release includes forward-looking statements on our current expectations and projections about future events. In some cases forward-looking statements can be identified by terminology such as "may," "should," "potential," "continue," "expects," "anticipates," "intends," "plans," "believes," "estimates," and similar expressions. These statements are based upon current beliefs, expectations and assumptions and are subject to a number of risks and uncertainties, many of which are difficult to predict. The information in this release is provided only as of the date of this release, and we undertake no obligation to update any forward-looking statements contained in this release based on new information, future events, or otherwise, except as required by law.

University of Manitoba Study

Youngevity International (YGYI) Announces Results of Youngevity Research Studies Performed by the Richardson Center for Functional Foods and Nutraceuticals – University of Manitoba

San Diego, CA – May 28, 2014 – Youngevity International, Inc. (OTCQX: YGYI) (www.YGYI.com), a global direct marketer of lifestyle and nutritional products and gourmet coffee, announced today the exciting results of research studies performed at the prestigious Richardson Center for Functional Foods and Nutraceuticals (RCFFN) at the University of Manitoba (www.rcffn.ca).

The RCFFN is one of the most advanced bioprocessing and product development facilities in the world that focuses on the research, discovery, and development of innovative functional foods and nutraceuticals. The research team at the RCFFN evaluated the safety and health benefits of the following Youngevity signature products; Beyond Tangy Tangerine 2.0 and the Healthy Start Pak 2.0, which consists of the Beyond Tangy Tangerine 2.0, Beyond Osteo Fx 2.0, and Ultimate Essential Fatty Acids.

The study was overseen by Dr. Peter Jones, Director of the RCFFN and one of the world's foremost researchers in dietary and nutraceutical determinants in the control of fat, energy metabolism, and various other critical health issues. Additionally, the study was conducted by Dr. Ramprasath Vanu Ramkumar, Adjunct Professor and Research Associate for the Department of Human Nutritional Sciences at the University of Manitoba.

"When initially developing the study outline for Youngevity, it was critical to investigate the important areas where the products could be of benefit and demonstrate a high level of safety, I believe we have accomplished that, these were very well thought out studies," said Dr. Peter Jones, RCFFN Director.

Youngevity Research Study Results:

Safety: RCFFN tested various levels of organ functions and metabolism to demonstrate the safety of Beyond Tangy Tangerine 2.0, Beyond Osteo Fx 2.0, and Ultimate Essential Fatty Acids. The biochemical indicators and measurement showed normal functioning and metabolism of the liver,

kidneys, and heart after supplementation with Beyond Tangy Tangerine 2.0 and the Healthy Start Pak 2.0 demonstrate no adverse reactions to these organs.

Weight Loss: Consumption of the Beyond Tangy Tangerine 2.0 as well as the Healthy Start Pak 2.0 significantly reduced the absolute weights of White Adipose Tissue (WAT) as well as WAT weight percentage of whole body weight. The study showed a significant reduction in adipose tissue weight and body fat mass.

Bone Health: Significant reductions in plasma concentrations of Alkaline Phosphatase, ALKP, an enzyme that promotes breakdown of bone were observed along with increases in concentrations of the bone building minerals, calcium and phosphorus.

Support for Normal Inflammatory Response: Inflammation was induced in the animal models by feeding them a high fat and sugar diet that triggers the Interleukin-6 inflammatory marker. After supplementation with both the Beyond Tangy Tangerine 2.0 and Healthy Start Pak 2.0 a significant reduction of the inflammatory marker was observed demonstrating support for normal inflammatory responses when placed under stressful conditions.

"It's very important that studies such as these are done in a unbiased, highly respected, academic setting. Consumers can feel confident in the results of these studies because of the "arms length" relationship that RCFFN had with Youngevity, we reported everything we found," said Dr. Ramprasath Vanu Ramkumar, University of Manitoba Associate Professor.

"Building on the previous research Youngevity performed with Clemson University, the RCFFN study results further substantiate the incredible potential value and benefit our consumers can receive with the Youngevity products. Youngevity is one of the few companies that provide such comprehensive research along with their products and we are proud to do so," said Sanjeev Javia, Youngevity Scientific Advisory Board Member.

"For over 15 years, Youngevity has been committed to science backed nutrition and providing the highest quality nutrients, dietary supplements, and wellness products to our distributors and customers," said Steve Wallach, CEO and Chairman of Youngevity. "We are very excited and proud of the research results achieved on our signature products by the world-class researchers at the prestigious Richardson Center for Functional Foods and Nutraceuticals. The research studies performed on our products at Clemson University in 2012 and the University of Manitoba provide further support for the value and health benefits that we believe can be obtained from our products and Youngevity's dedication to research and innovation."

About Youngevity International Inc.

THE NUTRITION REVOLUTION

Youngevity International Inc., (OTCQX: YGYI) (www.YGYI.com) is a fast-growing, innovative, multi-dimensional company that offers a wide range of consumer products and services, primarily through person-to-person selling relationships that comprise a "network of networks." The Company also is a vertically-integrated producer of the finest coffees for the commercial, retail and direct sales channels. The Company was formed after the merger of Youngevity Essential Life Sciences (www.youngevity.com) and Javalution Coffee Company in the summer of 2011. The company was formerly known as AL International, Inc. and changed its name to Youngevity International Inc. in July 2013.

Safe Harbor Statement

This release includes forward-looking statements on our current expectations and projections about future events, including our continued growth. In some cases forward-looking statements can be identified by terminology such as "may," "should," "potential," "continue," "expects," "anticipates," "intends," "plans," "believes," "estimates," "encouraged" and similar expressions. The forward looking statements include statements regarding our expected future growth, international expansion and improved profit. These statements are based upon current beliefs, expectations and assumptions and are subject to a number of risks and uncertainties, many of which are difficult to predict such as our ability to continue our financial performance. The information in this release is provided only as of the date of this release, and we undertake no obligation to update any forward-looking statements contained in this release based on new information, future events, or otherwise, except as required by law.

Salt, 3/4/2015

Study Title Cutaneous Na⁺ Storage
Strengthens the Antimicrobial Barrier Function of the Skin and
Boosts Macrophage-Driven Host Defense

Jonathan Jantsch, Valentin Schatz, Diana Friedrich,
Agnes Schröder, Christoph Kopp, Isabel Siegert, Andreas
Maronna, David Wendelborn, Peter Linz, Katrina J. Binger,
Matthias Gebhardt, Matthias Heinig, Patrick Neubert, Fabian
Fischer, Stefan Teufel, Jean-Pierre David, Clemens Neufert,
Alexander Cavallaro, Natalia Rakova, Christoph Küper,
Franz-Xaver Beck, Wolfgang Neuhofer, Dominik N. Muller,
Gerold Schuler, Michael Uder, Christian Bogdan, Friedrich C.
Luft,

Jens Titze Co-first author

http://dx.doi.org/10.1016/j.cmet.2015.02.003

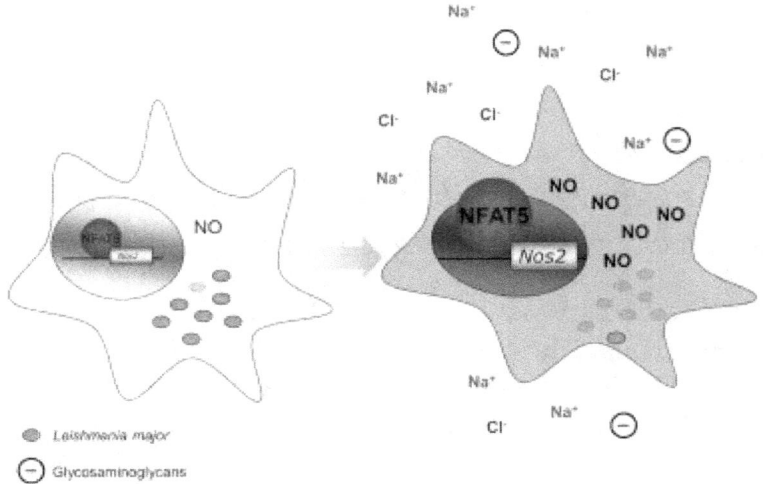

Highlights

- Na⁺ (sodium ion) accumulates at site of bacterial skin infections in humans and in mice

- Salt boosts classical macrophage (MΦ) activation and wards off infection

- Salt increases NOS2 activity in MΦ via p38/MAPK and NFAT5 signaling

- High-salt diet promotes skin Na⁺ storage and ameliorates cutaneous leishmaniasis

(Salt continued)

Summary

Immune cells regulate a hypertonic microenvironment in the skin; however, the biological advantage of increased skin Na⁺ concentrations is unknown.

We found that Na⁺ accumulated at the site of bacterial skin infections in humans and in mice.

We used the protozoan parasite LEISHMANIA MAJOR as a model of skin-prone macrophage infection to test the hypothesis that skin-Na⁺ storage facilitates antimicrobial host defense.

Activation of macrophages in the presence of high NaCl concentrations modified epigenetic markers and enhanced p38 mitogen-activated protein kinase (p38/MAPK)-dependent nuclear factor of activated T cells 5 (NFAT5) activation.

This high-salt response resulted in elevated type-2 nitric oxide synthase (NOS2)-dependent NO production and improved LEISHMANIA MAJOR control.

Finally, we found that increasing Na⁺ content in the skin by a high-salt diet boosted activation of macrophages in a NFAT5-dependent manner and promoted cutaneous antimicrobial defense. We suggest that the hypertonic microenvironment could serve as a barrier to infection.

TEXT

You can find the entire study, including copious diagrams and the experimental methodology, here:

http://www.cell.com/cell-metabolism/fulltext/S1550-4131%2815%2900055-8

RELATED WORK ON SALT

New England Journal of Medicine, August 2014

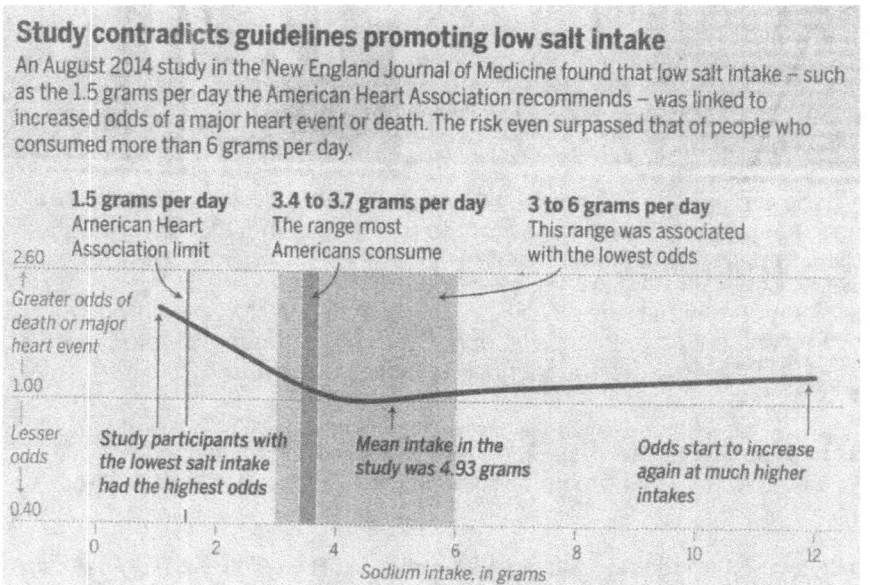

Study contradicts guidelines promoting low salt intake

An August 2014 study in the New England Journal of Medicine found that low salt intake – such as the 1.5 grams per day the American Heart Association recommends – was linked to increased odds of a major heart event or death. The risk even surpassed that of people who consumed more than 6 grams per day.

1.5 grams per day
American Heart Association limit

3.4 to 3.7 grams per day
The range most Americans consume

3 to 6 grams per day
This range was associated with the lowest odds

2.60

Greater odds of death or major heart event

1.00

Lesser odds

0.40

Study participants with the lowest salt intake had the highest odds

Mean intake in the study was 4.93 grams

Odds start to increase again at much higher intakes

0   2   4   6   8   10   12
Sodium intake, in grams

This graph is reprinted from the San Diego Union Tribune,

March 4, 2015.

Important points:

1. The American Heart Association AHA recommends limiting salt intake to only 1.5 grams a day.

    The study found that this limitation <u>Increased</u> the risk of a major heart event of death By 75%.

2. Despite the AHA recommendation, most Americans consume 3.4 to 3.7 grams per day, more than twice what the AHA recommends.

3. The lowest incidence of major heart events and death occurred among people consuming 4.5 grams of salt a day.

4.   Even at a massive 12 grams a day, the risk of a major heart event or death is only increased by 25%.

5. The graph has a conclusion. 3 to 6 grams of salt a day is associated with Lowest Odds of a major heart event or death.

The newspaper article also makes statements like these:

"It's the latest chapter in research exploring the role of salt in the human body, a story that keeps growing more complicated.

"That's also true of fat and cholesterol, which have long been highlighted as causes of poor health. This original stance has been undermined by recent research that tells a more complex story than what has been advanced through decades of government health advisories.

"In February (2015), the federal government said it would drop its caution about cholesterol intake.

"Also last month (2/15) previous warnings to cut dietary fat were undercut by a new report.

"Last year (2014) multiple studies found that predicted benefits from restricting sodium intake weren't justified. One of these studies concluded that the federal government's recommended levels of sodium intake actually could be low.

"In short, the latest science emphasizes that old notions about fat, cholesterol and salt are far too simplistic for a complex system such as human metabolism. It also reflects a growing contention among some scientists that medical and dietary standards should be customized for each patient or particular groups of patients, not for an entire nation."

As further evidence, Jens Titze said that one patient with an infected leg developed a salt buildup that didn't appear in the uninfected leg.

Regarding the salt limit of 1.5 grams a day, in 2013, the Institute of Medicine wrote, *"Overall, the committee found that both the quantity and quality of relevant studies to be less than optimal."*

That is about as stern a rebuke as one finds in the self-congratulating medical science community.

NUTRITION REVOLUTION

The Institute of Medicine went on to state, *"...there wasn't enough evidence to conclude that lowering sodium intake below 2.3 grams per day would increase or decrease the risk of cardiovascular disease or death in the general population."*

Noted Scripps Clinic cardiologist in la Jolla, CA, Dr. Eric Topel underlined these findings, adding that *"Some people are exquisitely sensitive to salt intake, while others are remarkably resistant."* He continues, stating that everyone is quite different and each person needs a different diet, including a different level of salt intake.

It's almost like Topel is parroting Dr. Joel Wallach, who has said for more than a decade, *"Salt to taste,"* as well as this book which declares that your body, tongue and palate will tell you EXACTLY how much salt is best for you.

BIBLIOGRAPHY

1. Study and article debunking low salt limitations.

http://www.cell.com/cell-metabolism/fulltext/S1550-4131
%2815%2900055-8   (all in one line)

http://utsandiego/saltinfection

2. Article and transcript about no longer restricting cholesterol.
     (citation coming soon)

3. Joel Wallach and Ma Lan: Dead Doctors Don't Lie, Wellness Publications. CD and DVD also available.

4. Will David Mitchell: The Seduction of DoctoRx, Intellectual Properties SD.

5. Robert Kobarg and Will David Mitchell, Essential Nutrition, Intellectual Properties SD. CD set available.

6. Joel Wallach and Ma Lan: Hell's Kitchen, Wellness Publications. CD available.

7. Joel Wallach and Ma Lan: Epigenetics, Death of the Genetic Theory of Disease Transmission, Wellness Publications.

8. Joel Wallach and Ma Lan: Energy Crisis, Wellness Publications. CD available.

9. Joel Wallach and Ma Lan: Let's Play Doctor, Wellness Publications.

10. Joel Wallach and Ma Lan: Let's Play Herbal Doctor, Wellness Publications.

11. Joel Wallach and Ma Lan: Rare Earths: Forbidden Cures, Wellness Publications. CD available

12. Joel Wallach and Ma Lan: God Bless America, Wellness Publications.

13. Joel Wallach and Ma Lan: Black Gene Lies, Wellness Publications. CD available.

14. Joel Wallach and Ma Lan: Immortality, Wellness Publications. CD available.

15. Valerie Nielson: Gluten-Free and Loving It, Wellness Publications.

WHERE TO FIND THIS BOOK

Softcover, color version available from Amazon.

Electronic versions available:

- Kindle,

- PDF,

Thank you kindly for your time spent reading. I pray for your health.

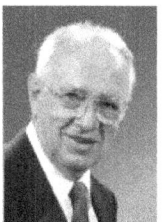

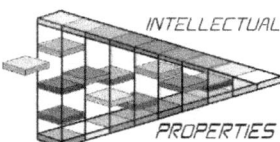 Nutritionist
858-538-2911, 9-9 Pacific Time.

Published by Intellectual Properties SD.

Published by Intellectual Properties SD.

Produced and printed in the USA.

www.ingramcontent.com/pod-product-compliance
Lightning Source LLC
Chambersburg PA
CBHW081345280526
45788CB00009B/2778